Breast Cancer

Journey to Recovery

Carol Noll Hoskins, PhD, RN, FAAN, is Professor of Nursing at New York University, where she served as Director of the Program in Research and Theory Development in Nursing Science (1985–1990). Her research focuses on adjustment of the family to illness, repeated-measures designs, and psychometrics. She is the author of two measures of interactive behaviors in the partner relationship, *The Partner Relationship Inventory* and *The Dominance-Accommodation Scale.*

Professor Hoskins was Principal Investigator for a longitudinal study of psychosocial adjustment among women with breast cancer and their partners (1990–1994). The findings were used to develop a four-part instructional videotape series, *Journey to Recovery: For Women with Breast Cancer and their Partners.* The phase-specific content is applicable to the diagnostic, postsurgical, adjuvant therapy, and ongoing recovery periods. She is currently the Principal Investigator on phase III of the program of research, a randomized clinical trial to study the effectiveness of standardized education by videotape, telephone counseling, or a combination of the two interventions.

Judith Haber, PhD, APRN, CS, FAAN, is a family therapist in private practice in Stamford, CT and Professor and Director of the Master's and Post-Master's Certificate Programs in the Division of Nursing at New York University. She is also a founding partner in a professional image consulting firm, Image Care Associates. Dr. Haber was formerly Professor and Director of the Department of Nursing at the College of Mount Saint Vincent, Riverdale, New York.

Dr. Haber earned her baccalaureate degree in nursing, cum laude, from Adelphi University and her master's and doctoral degrees from New York University. She earned a Certificate of Advanced Achievement in Family Therapy from the Center for Family learning, New Rochelle, New York and is certified by the American Nurses Credentialing Center as a Clinical Specialist in Adult Psychiatric-Mental Health Nursing.

Dr. Haber is internationally recognized as a clinician and educator in psychiatric-mental health nursing. She has received two AJN Book of the Year awards for her classic textbook *Comprehensive Psychiatric Nursing,* recently published in its 5th edition and translated into Spanish and French. Dr. Haber is also co-editor of *Nursing Research: Methods, Critical Appraisal and Utilization,* now in its 4th edition, translated into German and Italian, and recipient of a 1994 AJN Book of the Year Award.

Wendy C. Budin, PhD, RN, C, is Associate Professor of Nursing and Program Director of the Lamaze International Childbirth Educator Certification Program at Seton Hall University. She received the first NJ Breast Cancer Visiting Research Scholar Fellowship, awarded by the NJ State Commission on Cancer Research, 1996, to work with Dr. Carol Noll Hoskins on the video project *Journey to Recovery: For Women with Breast Cancer and Their Partners.* Dr. Budin's research "Psychosocial Adjustment to Breast Cancer in Unmarried Women" was funded by a grant from the American Nurses Foundation, and she was named the 1994 ANF, Barbara A. Given, Scholar. For this research, she also received the 1997 Sigma Theta Tau International Regional Research Dissertation Award. Dr. Budin is also coauthor of the 6th edition of *Notter's Essentials of Nursing Research* (Springer Publishing Co.).

Breast Cancer

Journey to Recovery

Carol Noll Hoskins, PhD, RN, FAAN
Judith Haber, PhD, APRN, CS, FAAN
and **Wendy Budin,** PhD, RN, C

SP Springer Publishing Company

Springer Publishing Company, Inc.
536 Broadway
New York, NY 10012-3955

This book is an adaptation of a set of four videos created by
Carol Noll Hoskins and the Division of Nursing, New York
University. The video set, *Journey to Recovery: For Women with
Breast Cancer and Their Partners,* was produced by Euro Pacific
Film and Video Productions, Inc. It is distributed by Films for
the Humanities and Sciences in Princeton, New Jersey. The
videos are also available from Springer Publishing Co.

Acquisitions Editor: Ruth Chasek
Production Editor: Pamela Lankas
Cover design by Susan Hauley

01 02 03 04 05 / 5 4 3 2 1

Library of Congress Cataloging-in-Publication Data

Hoskins, Carol Noll.
    Breast cancer : journey to recovery / Carol Noll Hoskins,
    Judith Haber, and Wendy Budin.
        p. cm.
    Includes bibliographical references and index.
    ISBN 0-8261-1392-3 (softcover)
    1. Breast—Cancer—Popular works.   I. Haber, Judith.
II. Budin, Wendy C.   III. Title.

RC280.B8 H667 2001
362.1'9699449—dc21

                                                    00-046388

Printed in the United States of America by Capital City Press, USA

Contents

Preface   *vii*

1   Coping With a Diagnosis of Breast Cancer   **1**
    Facts About Breast Cancer   2
    Methods for Diagnosing Breast Cancer   4
    Surgical Treatments   10
    Understanding Perceptions, Emotions, and Concerns   16
    Recognizing and Managing Stress   17
    Identifying Health Care Resources   20
    Knowledge Review   23

2   Recovering From Surgery   **28**
    Recognizing Feelings After Surgery   29
    Promoting Physical Healing   29
    Strategies to Promote Psychological Recovery   33
    Managing Changes in Family and Social Roles   39
    Summary   41
    Knowledge Review   42

3   Understanding Adjuvant Therapy   **47**
    Types of Adjuvant Therapies and Indications   48
    Getting More Information on Treatment   54
    Enhancing Physical and Emotional Health   56
    Avoiding Infections or Illness   58
    Maintaining Good Nutrition   58
    Planning Frequent Periods of Rest With a Balance of Activity   59
    Managing Menopause-Like Symptoms   60
    Other Management Strategies   61
    Knowledge Review   64

4 Ongoing Recovery   **70**
  Recognizing Emotional Concerns and Challenges   71
  Maintaining a Support Network   77
  Developing a Plan for Ongoing Medical Care   82
  Knowledge Review   87

**5 A Program of Research: Breast Cancer Education,   91
    Counseling, and Adjustment Among Patients
    and Partners**
  Phase I: Preliminary Study   92
  Phase II: Development of the Structured   94
    Educational Intervention
  Phase III: Pilot Study and Start-Up of a Randomized   95
    Clinical Trial
  Interventions   96

References   *99*

Appendix: Cancer Resources in the United States   *103*

Answers to "Test Your Knowledge" Questions   *107*

Index   *111*

Preface

The publication of *Breast Cancer: Journey to Recovery* represents a tribute to all women with breast cancer and their partners. Breast cancer affects women of all ages, races, ethnicities, socioeconomic strata, and geographic areas. It continues to rob families of mothers, grandmothers, sisters, wives, and partners. This year alone approximately 183,000 women in the United States will be diagnosed with breast cancer, and more than 41,000 will succumb to the disease (American Cancer Society, 2000).

Although adjustment to breast cancer presents an overwhelming challenge to women, or men, who are afflicted with the diagnosis, as well as those who are close to them, of special note is the impact of the breast cancer diagnosis on the partner, whether the partner is a marital or non-marital significant other.

The seminal 4-year research study by Dr. Carol Hoskins of how 121 couples dealt with the diagnosis and treatment of breast cancer provided data for the development of a unique, award-winning, four-part educational video series, *Journey to Recovery: For Women With Breast Cancer and Their Partners*. By offering essential evidence-based information, strategies for skills development, and psychosocial support, the videos were designed to help women and men cope with the severe stress of each unique phase of the breast cancer experience. This book is an adaptation of the video series. Written for professional health care providers as well as consumers of health care, the book guides professionals and consumers alike through each phase of the breast cancer diagnosis, treatment, and recovery trajectory. Chapter 1 helps couples cope with the breast cancer diagnosis. Chapter 2 walks couples through recovering from surgery. Chapter 3 tackles the issues of adjuvant therapy, that is, radiation, chemotherapy, and hormone therapy. Chapter 4 emphasizes the importance of the ongoing recovery process. Chapter 5 provides the reader with an overview of Dr. Carol Hoskins' seminal Patterns of Adjustment research study. A content outline is provided with chapters 1 through 4, which can be used as a helpful review of key points for patients and professionals. Each outline is followed by a "Test Your Knowledge" series of questions.

Throughout the book, readers meet real couples dealing with breast cancer and learn how they have coped with this experience. They also meet noted health professionals who provide important advice and information about meeting the challenges of coping with breast cancer. Readers also obtain important information about essential community-based and internet breast cancer resources. Health professionals will have the wealth of information contained in *Breast Cancer: Journey to Recovery*, to use when teaching and counseling women with breast cancer and their partners how to cope effectively with each phase of the diagnosis, treatment, and recovery trajectory of the breast cancer experience. This book would not have been possible without the generous commitment of time and willingness to share with others an intimate, life altering health experience. Our thanks to those women and their partners, Linda and Bob, Carol and George, and Nellie, who graciously chose to reveal their lived experience so that others might benefit from their wisdom. Special thanks go to renowned breast surgeon Dr. Roy Ashikari and medical oncologist Dr. Abraham Mittleman whose oncology expertise lends such credibility and vigor to the book. Special recognition also goes to Lisa Moss of Euro-Pacific Film and Video Productions for the loving care with which she edited and refined the video script that provided the foundation of this project. Our sincere gratitude goes to the artist, George McNeil, who provided the original art for the illustrations in both the book and videotape series. His generous contribution of talent and time are deeply appreciated. We also would like to thank those who as Doctoral Fellows contributed so much to the richness of this project, Dr. Deborah Sherman, Frances Cartwright-Alcarese, and Mildred Ortu Kowalski, as well as our Research Assistant, Joan Panke. Finally, we are grateful to our families whose loving support, patience, and understanding helped make this exciting project a reality.

Coping With a Diagnosis of Breast Cancer

Linda is a breast cancer survivor who has undergone breast reconstruction following removal of her breast. Bob is Linda's husband.

LINDA: *Death. I think that's your first reaction to that word "cancer", no matter what. And it wasn't a word I expected to hear so it, makes it even worse, you know, thinking about your kids, you know, my life, just all of it kind of passing before you when you hear that word. Fright.*

BOB: *I didn't know what to really do except be there for her, do whatever I could, but I didn't know, I was afraid.*

Carol is a breast cancer survivor with a lumpectomy. George is Carol's husband.

CAROL: *Why did this happen? What did I do? Why, why me? I was very angry.*

GEORGE: *I didn't believe it was malignant was my first thought. My mind wouldn't allow me to believe it was that.*

Nellie is a breast cancer survivor with a lumpectomy. She is not married.

NELLIE: *Initially it was a shock. It wasn't that I was anticipating anything that I had it. It started out as a pain in my right breast. I never thought that it was anything close to cancer. If anything, I suspected it was a cyst.*

Women who have had a diagnosis of breast cancer and their partners experience many of these very same feelings and have many questions. How will I cope? How can I make the best choice for treatment? How can I assure that I will get the best care? This book will help answer some of these questions.

Since breast cancer is a health problem one of eight American women may experience, it has received much attention in the media. You probably already know some of the facts about breast cancer, but it is only when one's life is directly affected by an illness that one begins a search for the most current information. The way in which women and their partners deal with diagnosis and treatment of breast cancer was studied recently by nurse researchers at New York University. The information from the study provides the content for this book.

The purpose of the study and this book is to help women with breast cancer, their families, and their health care providers to:

- learn about types and stages of breast cancer
- understand surgical treatments
- identify concerns and perceptions
- recognize and manage stress
- identify health care resources
- learn how and where to seek support

FACTS ABOUT BREAST CANCER

Let's begin with an understanding of some of the facts about breast cancer. Cancer is an abnormal growth of cells. The cells divide more than they should and form lumps known as tumors. Cancerous tumors may interfere with normal tissue.

Cells may break away from the original tumor and travel to other parts of the body by way of the blood stream or a circulatory system known as the lymph system. Lymph nodes are small glands located in the armpit and serve as a kind of block to the cells spreading to other parts of the body. By beginning treatment as soon as possible, one can catch the cancer before it spreads.

Despite advances in detection and treatment, breast cancer statistics remain daunting; breast cancer afflicts women of all ages, races, ethnicities, socioeconomic strata, and geographic areas. Breast cancer is expected to continue as the most common cancer diagnosed in women (American Cancer Society, 1998, 2000). Estimates for the number of new cases of breast cancer in women for the year 2000 are 183,000 (American Cancer Society, 2000). Mortality estimates have begun to decrease, however, and in the year 2000 estimates are 41,000 (American Cancer Society, 2000). The basis for the decrease in mortality estimates since 1994 has been attributed to early detection and improved treatments (Parker, Tong, Bolden, & Wingo, 1997), whereas an apparent increase in incidence until recently was also attributed to early detection (Hortobagyi, 1993). Although more than 90% of those afflicted with breast cancer survive for five years or longer, they often feel extremely uncertain about the future, which affects how well they and their families adjust both emotionally and physically.

The diagnosis of breast cancer begins with a physical examination and a mammogram, usually recommended for women over 40 who have a standard visit for breast cancer screening (Hortobagyi, 1993). Mammography quality has improved in the past 10 to 15 years. Also patients' awareness of breast cancer, thanks to the media, has increased. Therefore more patients have a mammography, clinical examination, and perhaps perform breast self-examination.

LINDA: *One of the risk factors that I probably had that I found out later was the fact that I didn't have a biological child until I was in my late thirties, and that is a risk factor.*

CAROL: *I have a couple of aunts who had cancer later in life but not breast cancer. So there was not a high visit factor of family history. I have 5 brothers and 3 sisters and all are very healthy. My mother's healthy, and it just totally shocked me.*

NELLIE: *I don't have a family history of breast cancer, so it was a total shock.*

Are all women at risk, or are some women more likely to get breast cancer? There are some factors that are associated with placing a woman more or less at risk. These factors might include increasing age, a family history of breast cancer, age at birth of first child, say, well into her thirties, never given birth, early menstrual period, late menopause, high-fat diet, obesity, high alcohol consumption, or a high dose of radiation to the chest (see Table 1.1). It is not known whether the prolonged use of oral contraceptives or estrogen replacement therapy is a risk factor for breast cancer.

Before we get to the diagnosis and treatment options for breast cancer, let's get a clear view of the structure of the breast. Breasts are mainly fatty tissue with glands that can produce milk. The glands of the breast are known as lobules that are connected to the nipple by slender tubes known as ducts (see Figure 1.1). Most breast cancers begin in the ducts.

METHODS FOR DIAGNOSING BREAST CANCER

If a lump is detected through mammography, its size and the nature of its growth must be assessed. With a suspicious lump or breast change, a breast biopsy probably will be recommended. A fine-needle aspiration biopsy in the doctor's office involves the placement of a very fine needle in the suspicious area, and a few cells are removed for examination under a microscope (see Figure 1.2). The core needle biopsy is used on a palpable lesion—something that a physician or a surgeon can feel and stick a needle in.

Stereotactic breast biopsy is the latest technologic advance in diagnosing breast cancer, and it's used on suspicious lesions that are detected on the mammogram. It's done to detect whether the lesion is benign or malignant.

In this procedure, Elaine Kloos, RN, MSN, OCN, Program Director of the Hunterdon Regional Cancer Program in New Jersey explains, "A computer is used for guidance to locate the lesion. Once x-rays are taken, and with very accurate pinpoint decision making with the computer, the needle is placed in the breast, and 3 to 5 samples are taken. They're sent to pathology for histological analysis, and typically the results can be given to a woman in 24 to 48 hours."

The treatment of breast cancer depends on a number of factors, including the type of cancer (see Table 1.2). Noninvasive breast cancer, or *carcinoma in situ,* means confined to one site or place. These kinds of cancer usually do not spread. When noninvasive cancer is located in a lobe, it is considered a marker of increased risk because it may not be seen on mammography or found in a biopsy that is otherwise negative.

TABLE 1.1   Risk Factors

- Increasing age
- History of breast cancer
- Family history of breast cancer
- Age at birth of first child
- Never given birth
- Early menstrual period
- Late menopause
- High fat diet
- Obesity
- High alcohol consumption
- High dose radiation to chest
- Oral contraceptives or estrogen replacement therapy may be a risk

Invasive or infiltrating cancer moves beyond the original site and invades other parts of the breast. Infiltrating ductal carcinoma accounts for about 80% of invasive breast cancers. Infiltrating lobular cancers account for 10 to 15% of invasive breast cancers.

When a woman has a breast biopsy, the cells are examined by a pathologist to make a diagnosis and to provide information on the stage of the breast cancer.

TABLE 1.2   Types of Breast Cancer

Noninvasive Breast Cancers:
    Ductal Carcinoma in Situ
- Most common type of noninvasive breast cancer
- Confined to ducts
- Does not spread through walls of the ducts

    Lobular Carcinoma in Situ
- Begins in lobules, but does not penetrate lobule walls
- Marker of increased risk of invasive cancer in either breast

Invasive Breast Cancers:
    Infiltrating Ductal Carcinoma
- 80% of all breast cancers
- Starts in duct
- Invades the breast's fatty tissues

    Infiltrating Lobular Carcinoma
- 10% to 15% of invasive breast cancers
- Starts in glands
- Can spread

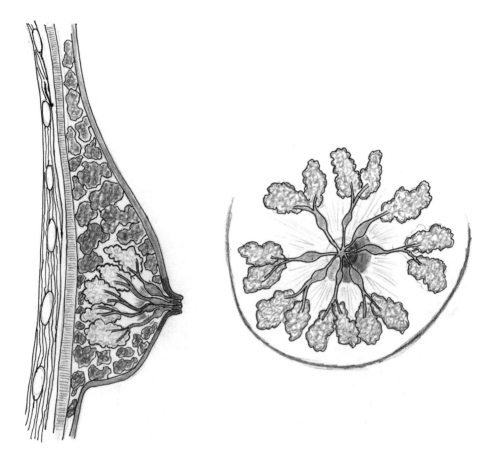

FIGURE 1.1   Appearance of a healthy breast.

The four important things to know about breast cancer are:

- the size and extent of the primary tumor
- whether cancer cells have spread to the lymph nodes
- whether cells have spread to other parts of the body
- the characteristics of the cancer cells as determined by microscopic, or histological examination

LINDA: *I did go to a surgeon who said to me, "I wouldn't worry about it. It moves, it hurts. Those are usually the type that are absolutely fine." But at that point I had lived with this fear now for a couple of months and I said to him, "You*

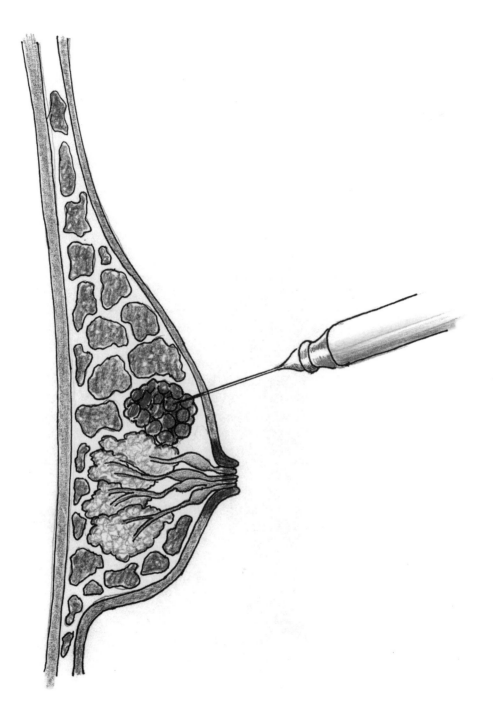

FIGURE 1.2   Fine-needle aspiration biopsy.

7

know what? I just want it out. I don't want to watch it. I don't want anything, I just want it out." And so I went to have a lumpectomy at that point. . . . And the doctor, right up until after the surgery, told me everything was fine. And it was only subsequently when no one was getting back to me, I kept calling and asking, "What are the results? What are the results?" And I wasn't getting any answers. They kept putting me off. And I had to leave and go on a business trip which, you know, sometimes things happen for a reason. I happened to be down in New York near my original doctor, my breast specialist down here, and finally after hot pursuit the doctor did call me and told me over the phone that it was bad news, that it was cancer. And it was hard.

The staging of the cancer is done by histologic and other examinations of the tumor after it has been removed. Let's clarify more of what we mean about the stages of cancer. In Table 1.3 you see stages 0 to 4. Knowing these stages is extremely important when making a decision about how to proceed with treatment.

Stage 0 means the cancer is confined, usually in the ducts. Stage 1 means the cancer is localized, without spreading to the lymph nodes. Stage 2 refers to limited spread to local tissue or lymph nodes. Stage 3 indicates a larger tumor with spread to the lymph nodes. And stage 4 means cancer has spread to other parts of the body by way of the lymph nodes (see Figure 1.3).

CAROL:　. . . *When I had my mammogram they found calcification that looked suspicious, but I really didn't think it was cancer. I knew there was a chance, so I went in for the biopsy, and they had planned to do the surgery if it was in fact cancer. And that's what they did, so I didn't know until I was in the operating room and I was doped up.*

TABLE 1.3　Stages of Breast Cancer

Stage 0—Cancer is confined
Stage 1—Localized cancer
Stage 2—Limited spread
Stage 3—Larger tumor, with spread to lymph nodes
Stage 4—Cancer spread to other parts of the body

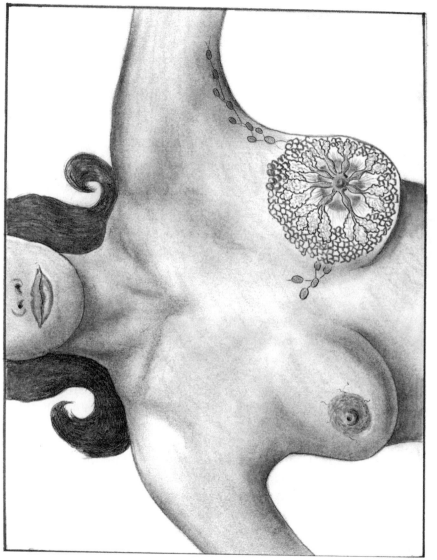

FIGURE 1.3 Illustration of how cancer cells spread by lymph nodes.

SURGICAL TREATMENTS

We know that early intervention is critical for the most successful treatment of breast cancer. But how does a woman and her partner decide what kind of surgery to have? Consider some of these factors.

Women today may be presented with a choice of surgery that either preserves the breast or surgery that removes the whole breast. The choice of surgery and follow-up treatments will depend on both the type of breast cancer and the stage. Other considerations are a woman's age, her overall health, and her willingness to accept certain side effects.

Let's talk first about the breast conservation approaches most often used for early stages of breast cancer.

With a lumpectomy, the tumor is removed, along with a margin of healthy tissue. Some lymph nodes are also removed from the arm pit (Figure 1.4). Dr. Roy Ashikari, a leading cancer surgeon and authority on breast cancer explains that "about 50% of early breast cancers are now treated by lumpectomy. Indications for a lumpectomy are (a) a single lesion in the breast; (b) the cancer is small—the ratio between the cancer itself and the size of the breast is very important."

Whether a woman has had a lumpectomy or mastectomy, her physicians need to know whether the cancer has spread to the lymph nodes in the arm pit, or axilla, a portal of entry for cancer cells to enter the blood stream and spread throughout the body. Either an axillary lymph node dissection or a sentinel lymph node biopsy is conducted. An axillary lymph node dissection involves a surgical incision in the axillary area under the arm. A sampling of lymph nodes is removed and examined microscopically for evidence of spread of cancer cells to the lymph nodes. A newer procedure, the sentinel lymph node biopsy, involves the sentinel node, the first lymph node into which the tumor drains, and the one most likely to contain cancer cells (Gross, 1998). A radioactive substance or blue dye is injected into the area around the breast tumor. Lymphatic vessels carry these materials into the sentinel node. The surgeon can either see the blue dye or detect the radioactivity with a Geiger counter. The surgeon makes a small incision in the axilla and cuts out the node for examination. If the sentinel node contains cancer, a lymph node dissection, removal of more lymph nodes in the axilla (armpit) is undertaken. If the sentinel

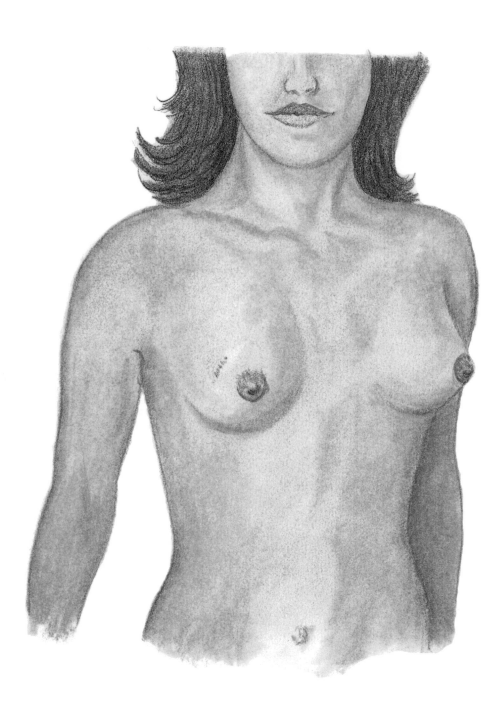

FIGURE 1.4   Illustration of a lumpectomy.

node is cancer free, the patient can avoid more lymph node surgery and the related side effects such as numbness, restricted arm movement, or lymphedema. The sentinel lymph node biopsy shows promise for reducing the number of unnecessary axillary lymph node dissections (Baron, 1999).

NELLIE: *I wanted to preserve my breast so I chose lumpectomy.*

Some earlier stage breast cancers may require a partial or segmental mastectomy. It takes not only the cancer, but a part of the breast tissue as well. Mastectomy used to be done for both big and small cancers, but now we know that often a lumpectomy has results that are as good as a mastectomy. That's why the incidence of lumpectomy or partial mastectomy has increased in the past few years.

When part of the breast is preserved, as in these procedures, there are usually follow-up treatments with moderate doses of radiation. Many studies indicate that if radiation is not given after a lumpectomy, the recurrence is higher than in patients receiving postoperative radiation. Therefore radiation therapy is routine after a lumpectomy.

In some situations, chemotherapy is administered in addition to radiation. These treatments are intended to eradicate any cancer cells that may remain after surgery. The treatments are not started until everything is healed following surgery.

CAROL: *I totally relied on my doctor. I totally trusted him. I felt confident. I had two girlfriends the same age as me who went to the same doctor and I went with them, as a matter of fact, for their visits before and I never thought I would be a patient. So I totally trusted him and if he said, "I want to do a mastectomy" that would have been fine. I just wanted the cancer gone. Whatever we have to do. I didn't care about disfigurement or anything like that. I just didn't want to have cancer.*

Some breast cancers may require what is known as a mastectomy, which is a nonbreast-conservation approach (see Table 1.4 and Figure 1.5). In other words, the breast is removed to effectively eliminate the cancer.

TABLE 1.4   Mastectomy Indications

- Tumor is greater than 4 cm
- Breast is very small
- Multiple cancers are in different parts of breast
- Calcifications in widely separated areas of the breast
- Pregnancy (follow-up radiation danger)
- Prior radiation to the breast

Doctors rely on certain indications before deciding to recommend removal of the breast. Mastectomy is usually indicated if the tumor is greater than 4 cm or the breast is very small; if there are multiple cancers in different parts of the breast; or if there are suspicious areas known as calcifications in widely separated areas of the breast. In addition, if the woman is pregnant, radiation follow-up may pose a danger, so removal of the breast may be a safer alternative for the baby and mother. And finally, prior radiation to the breast may present a problem.

With a simple or total mastectomy, only the breast is removed. This procedure is most appropriate for early breast cancers. The lymph nodes will either be left intact or sampled.

The second nonbreast-conserving procedure is a modified radical mastectomy. The breast, some lymph nodes in the armpit, and the lining over the chest muscles are removed .

A radical mastectomy is done only when the patient has a big tumor and many lymph nodes involved. Table 1.5 lists the different types of mastectomy.

> LINDA: *I was given the option of lumpectomy or mastectomy. One of the reasons why I chose not to have a lumpectomy, although I knew it was as effective, was because my lump was out near the nipple, so therefore they would have had to take off the nipple along with the lump and what's the point then? So that helped me make a decision to go with a mastectomy.*

If a woman has a mastectomy, she may want to consider breast reconstruction, which in recent years has become more common. Breast reconstruction reduces the changes in body appearance that occur as a result of surgery.

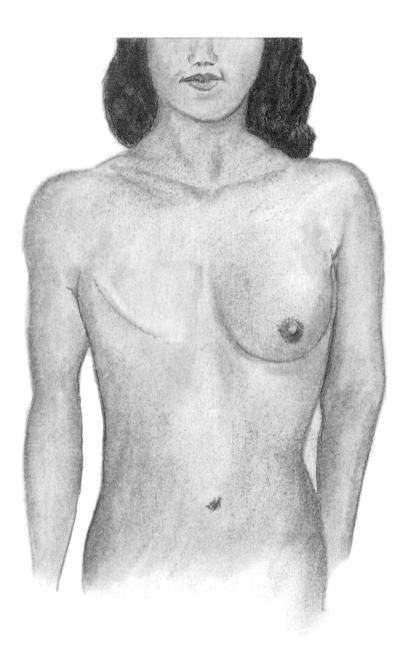

FIGURE 1.5   Illustration of a mastectomy.

TABLE 1.5   Types of Mastectomy

Total Mastectomy
- Only breast is removed
- For early breast cancers
- Lymph nodes may be left intact

Modified Radical Mastectomy
- Breast, lymph nodes in armpit, lining over chest muscles removed

Radical Mastectomy
- When breast cancer invades chest wall
- Breast, lymph nodes and some chest muscles removed

There are two types of reconstruction. It can be performed at the same time as the mastectomy or delayed until after the mastectomy. Immediate reconstruction can be done if the tumor is small, explains Dr. Roy Ashikari. "There is no reason to wait to do reconstruction at a later date because we can do it at the same time with one anesthesia, and also the patient wakes up to find a breast there. But these days not only the surgeon, but many other cancer specialists are involved." If reconstruction is done, such as an implant, and chemotherapy is given afterward, sometimes there are complications such as infection. "In these cases, I suggest that the patient wait until she finishes chemotherapy, or sometimes radiation therapy. Then we do the reconstruction," says Dr. Ashikari.

One method for breast reconstruction is a saline implant. An expander can be put in at the time of mastectomy, which slowly expands the implant area to make enough space. Then the expander is removed and the saline implant is inserted.

Another method of breast reconstruction is called a tram flap. The woman's own tissue is taken from the lower abdomen, back, or upper buttock and used as the implant.

The decision to have breast reconstruction really depends on what a woman prefers.

LINDA: *I was so lucky because my breast surgeon laid out the three reconstructive types of surgery that I could have and also strongly encouraged me to have simultaneous reconstruction because it would probably help me psychologically in the recovery process, to go through it a*

> *little quicker. . . . I guess, one of the things we discussed was there was saline, there was silicone, which at that time the controversy was just starting to brew about silicone, and then there was the tramflap, which would use a section of my own stomach to create a breast. . . . Since I had just had a baby I had enough stomach tissue there and it was nice, kind of, considering a tummy tuck, I was kind of losing one thing but kind of gaining something else. Umm, that appealed to me. . . . I then went back to Bob and talked about it. And I think we both felt that not having a foreign matter in my body was more appealing to both of us.*

BOB: *She was surrounded by a really great team of people who I had met before with her other lump, and I had basically educated myself on what some of the options were and I felt very confident in whatever she wanted to do.*

UNDERSTANDING PERCEPTIONS, EMOTIONS, AND CONCERNS

So far we've talked about the more technical and medical aspects of what a woman faces with a diagnosis of breast cancer. Feelings and attitudes about having breast cancer are powerful. They can help shape one's treatment and even one's eventual recovery.

Kathleen Conway, MSN, RN, CS, Clinical Director, who counsels cancer patients at the Center for Hope in Connecticut, explains, "It's a very devastating diagnosis for any woman at any age. And particularly, maybe it is even more for the younger woman with children. . . . If one's working, it's a threat to your economic security as well as your career. If you're a parent, it puts you in touch with your fears about your children and of course your spouse, how will he be?"

LINDA: *Just ice-cold fear. I felt like it was kind of surreal, like a movie. I couldn't be hearing this. . . . by the same token, you know, I wanted information then about what it was. You hear that word cancer, and your life kind of stands still.*

CAROL: *It was just horrible. The worst, the worst thing that could have happened. And it was a very traumatic experience for me. Very frightening. I thought I was, I was sure I was dying.*

NELLI: *It was a total shock because I couldn't believe that such a thing could happen to me.*

RECOGNIZE AND MANAGE STRESS

Symptoms of stress can be:

- changes in eating and sleeping
- difficulty focusing on work and family
- feeling nervous or anxious

For most women and their partners, finding a breast lump creates enormous fear—and stress. Managing that stress is vital to good health.

Although the New York University study (see more details about the study in the last chapter of this book) focused on couples, many findings may be applied to any woman diagnosed with breast cancer. The results were examined for women alone, as well as for partners alone. For example, partners described changes in their eating and sleeping patterns, difficulty focusing on their work and family responsibilities, and feeling very anxious. The symptoms of stress may affect either partner's ability to make important decisions. The management of stress is, therefore, extremely important to both partners' ultimate physical and emotional well-being.

LINDA: *I knew Bob would be with me all the way, no matter what it was, because we had been through a lot of difficult things in our life before. The one thing was, we always stuck together and we got through it, so I knew that was there. . . . a lot was going to fall on him since I had a new baby at home. Well, she was an infant. Two other 5-year-olds, and a lot was going to fall on him because the recovery process was going to be longer.*

BOB: *We had just moved into a new house that we built. So there's a lot of stress that goes along with that. Raising the boys, too. I started a business in Maine and then, you know, I was busy at work so that was stressful.*

LINDA: *For me, it actually became less stressful with every deci-sion. I think the most stressful thing was being in limbo. . . . And once I made my decision I felt in control. I felt we're taking action. I'm not in limbo and just allowing this to take over. I'm actively doing something about get-ting my body back to where it should be, and that relieved a lot of stress for me actually. . . . But I think people have to understand that they should take the time that they need to make the decision that is right for them. They have to look at their own individual circumstances and see what's right for them.*

Reducing stress is critical. It can help a woman concentrate on choosing the appropriate treatment and help her to focus on get-ting healthy.

It's important to gain a sense of control over events. According to Kathleen Conway, "It does reduce stress. We all know that when we have anxiety and we can take charge, our anxiety is reduced. When we can have some effect, we're not helpless in the face of illness. When we can look at the treatments, investigate them, or get someone else to do that information gathering for us and we look at it, we decide what we think is best rather than someone saying, 'This is what's best.' We feel a sense of control, we feel a sense of self-esteem, we don't feel helpless. And helplessness is what we think really does lead to depression and leads to perhaps not as good a course of illness."

Health and illness are life processes that change over time. The temporary loss of perfect health may be seen as an opportunity to cultivate an optimistic attitude to promote healing. Couples can do this in several ways.

- Develop a sense of control over events
- Cultivate an optimistic attitude
- Reduce tension through relaxation
- Send affirming messages; transform self-defeating, nega-tive feelings

A woman can discuss feelings with her partner, a close friend, or other person who will listen and permit her to be honest. Methods for stress reduction need to be developed. Letting go of tension through warm soothing baths, quiet moments listening to favorite music or relaxation tapes, or meditation are effective methods for getting in touch with the inner self and finding relaxation. Partners need to send affirming messages to one another.

Sometimes partners don't know what to do, and they feel helpless and they feel as scared as the person who's diagnosed with breast cancer. They also need some support so that they can have a way of talking about their fears, so that they don't always have to be the strong person, so that they can also let their guard down and talk about their fears.

In Kathleen Conway's experience, partners may be "trying to be there but sometimes they'll recognize that they've been working harder, that they've been staying at the office longer, that they've been distancing, and they've been doing it because they haven't known how to deal with their own intense feelings. . . . And that can also be a catalyst for helping the couple be close and actually share that scare or the emotions, which can bring them closer together in the relationship during this time of very intense crisis."

> CAROL: *I kept a diary and, I needed to talk to people who had been through the same thing. Like I would talk to my two girlfriends but they didn't go through the radiation so I wanted to talk to someone who went through the same thing that I went through and did well. I didn't want to hear anything negative.*

> GEORGE: *It was very difficult for me. I found that it was hard for me to really understand what Carol was going through. It was difficult for me to really feel what she was feeling. Umm, I know that I would say to her, "Gee, you look nice today" and it would backfire. "What does that mean? I looked lousy yesterday." So it didn't matter what I did at times. She was very, very on edge and very upset and difficult for me to understand.*

> CAROL: *I'm a nervous type. I tend to think the worst possible case, and George is just the opposite. He has a very strong nervous system. He's not a worrier. He's just, it*

happened, okay, it's over, get on with life. And that can be difficult because I needed to express it after it happened. It wasn't over for me. I still had to talk about all my feelings, so I found other friends and American Cancer Society people I spoke with who helped me through that; where George, it was over for him. But that's the way he is, and it's good for me. If he was the other type, if he was like me, it would feed my negativity when it comes to medical things.

IDENTIFYING HEALTH CARE RESOURCES

Once stress is under control, a woman can focus on selecting the best health care resources.

Barbara Rabinowitz, Director of Oncology Services, Meridian Health Services, gives the following advice on choosing a physician: "The relationship with a physician is really critical. There are really three major Cs. One is that the woman wants her physician to use every effort to go for *cure,* that she wants *control* of her symptoms and as much of the process as is possible, and also she wants *caring.* That is really such an important part that it often gets put to the side—women say this over and over again to researchers. Additionally, they want to know that they have good solid information from their physicians, information that isn't in the specific jargon of the physician. And they want to know that they can count on that relationship as they go forward through the process of diagnosis and then treatment."

If a woman has questions about the overall health care system of the hospital, the nurse, office staff, or a social worker can provide information about the health care system or insurance coverage. Nurses can help with information about routine hospital policies, payment procedures, and location of services. In most institutions, the preoperative tests, such as blood work, chest x-ray, and scans of bone and liver, if ordered by the doctor, may be performed on an outpatient basis.

Many women are admitted to the hospital on the day of their surgery and discharged within 1 to 4 days after surgery. It is often possible to coordinate the doctor's office visit with appointments to the laboratory or radiology departments so that valuable time and energy will not be lost in separate visits to the hospital. This is especially important after surgery when the energy level is not yet back to normal.

There are ways that people can try to create some control in their lives. For instance, Barbara Rabinovitz recommends that women make decisions about how they want their day and week to go, and what tasks they're going to do in the part of the day or week when they know they're going to feel better. A woman can decide when she wants her chemotherapy experience that week. She may choose Fridays because that gives her the weekend to try to recapture the sense of a more normal life.

Community Resources

It's important to explore community resources that can help. There are self-help groups for women with breast cancer that offer educational seminars and wellness programs.

Organizations such as the National Alliance of Breast Cancer in New York City, Reach to Recovery volunteers at local units of the American Cancer Society throughout the nation, and Why Me? that is located in Chicago are wonderful resources. They have women who have been through the breast cancer experience taking phone calls as well as having male partners of women who have been through the breast cancer experience taking partners' phone calls.

Seek Support From Health Care Providers, Family, Friends

A woman's experience of breast cancer touches the lives of all who care about her. As each one makes important decisions about treatment, comfort and support may be found by discussing feelings, concerns, and hopes with one's family doctor, partner, close family or friends. Many of the women in the study at New York University learned that talking with another woman who had been treated for breast cancer was very helpful. And men can also benefit from talking to other men whose partners had breast cancer. By openly expressing feelings and reaching out for answers, a woman and her partner can help themselves and be helped by others.

Active participation in breast cancer care will make all the difference in having as positive an experience as possible—from the point of diagnosis, through ongoing recovery, and living with breast cancer. Women should try to engage the support of family and friends and a health care team they trust. Sharing feelings, seeking information, and managing stress are valuable in adjusting to the challenging road ahead.

KNOWLEDGE REVIEW:
COPING WITH YOUR DIAGNOSIS

Content Outline

This section presents an outline of the content of the chapter. It may be used as a review of the key points, or as a helpful aid to health professionals in preparing educational material for patients.

I. Facts about breast cancer
  A. Abnormal growth of cells
    1. rapid cell division
    2. interfere with normal tissue
    3. may break away and travel to other parts of body
      a. blood stream
      b. lymph system
  B. Incidence of breast cancer
    1. second most common cancer among women
    2. rise in incidence may be related to early detection
    3. cause unknown
    4. risk factors
      a. increasing age
      b. history of breast cancer
      c. family history of breast cancer
      d. age at birth of first child
      e. never given birth
      f. early menstrual period
      g. late menopause
      h. high fat diet
      i. obesity
      j. high alcohol consumption
      k. high dose radiation to chest
  C. Structure of breast
    1. mainly fatty tissue with milk producing glands
      a. lobules
      b. ducts
  D. Methods for diagnosing breast cancer
    1. physical exam
    2. mammogram
    3. biopsy

      a. fine needle aspiration
      b. core needle biopsy
      c. stereotactic biopsy
  E. Types of breast cancer
    1. noninvasive
      a. ductal carcinoma in situ
      b. lobular carcinoma in situ
    2. invasive breast cancer
      a. infiltrating ductal carcinoma
      b. infiltrating lobular carcinoma
  F. Stages of breast cancer
    1. determinants
      a. size and extent of primary tumor
      b. spread to lymph nodes
      c. spread to other parts of body
    2. stages defined
      a. stage 0-cancer confined
      b. stage 1-localized cancer without spread to lymph nodes
      c. stage 2-limited spread to local tissue or lymph nodes
      d. stage 3-larger tumor with spread to lymph nodes
      e. stage 4-cancer spread to other body parts
II. Surgical treatment for breast cancer
  A. Factors affecting choice
    1. type of breast cancer
    2. stage of breast cancer
    3. age
    4. overall health
    5. personal preference
  B. Surgical treatment alternatives
    1. breast conserving approaches
      a. lumpectomy
      b. partial mastectomy
      c. follow-up treatment with radiation
      d. possible follow-up with chemotherapy
    2. nonbreast-conservation approaches
      a. simple or total mastectomy
      b. modified radical mastectomy
    3. breast reconstruction after mastectomy
      a. saline implant
      b. tram flap

III. Perceptions, emotions, and concerns
    A. Fear
    B. Disbelief
    C. Family concerns
    D. Work related concerns
    E. Need for information
IV. Recognizing and managing stress
    A. Signs of stress
        1. changes in eating and sleeping patterns
        2. difficulty focusing on work and family responsibilities
        3. feeling nervous or anxious
    B. Stress busters = active participation
        1. develop sense of control over events
        2. cultivate an optimistic attitude
        3. reduce tension through relaxation
            a. soothing baths
            b. quiet music or relaxation tapes
            c. meditation
        4. send affirming messages
            a. "We can cope"
            b. transform self-defeating, negative feelings
        5. keeping a journal or diary
        6. share feelings with family and others
V. Identifying health care resources
    A. Develop a positive relationship with physician
        1. concerns when selecting a physician
            a. cure
            b. control
            c. caring
        2. ask questions of health care providers
    B. Explore community resources
        1. breast cancer organizations
        2. self-help groups
        3. support groups
        4. educational programs
VI. Get support from a variety of sources
    A. Health care providers
    B. Family members
    C. Friends
    D. Others with similar experiences

Test Your Knowledge: Study Questions

Directions: Circle the letter corresponding to the correct response in each of the following.

1. Breast cancer is the second most common cancer among women.
    a. true
    b. false

2. There is no explanation for the apparent rise in the incidence of breast cancer.
    a. true
    b. false

3. Women with a family history of breast cancer are not at greater risk of developing breast cancer.
    a. true
    b. false

4. Most breast cancers begin in the ducts of the breast.
    a. true
    b. false

5. The stage of a tumor refers to the size.
    a. true
    b. false

6. A stereotactic needle biopsy uses a computer guided x-ray to pinpoint where to remove some cells from a suspicious lesion to detect if the lesion is benign or malignant.
    a. true
    b. false

7. Stage I indicates that the cancer is small and localized with no spread to the lymph nodes.
    a. true
    b. false

8. A disadvantage of a lumpectomy is that radiation follow-up treatment will be needed.
    a. true
    b. false

9. The decision whether to have breast reconstruction following mastectomy will depend on the woman's age.
    a. true
    b. false

10. Typical emotions experienced after the initial diagnosis of breast cancer include indifference followed by gradual adjustment.
    a. true
    b. false

11. There are a number of things a woman can do to decrease or manage the physical symptoms of stress.
    a. true
    b. false

12. It is recommended to share fears and concerns with a partner.
    a. true
    b. false

13. Medical expertise is the only important factor to consider when selecting a physician to treat breast cancer.
    a. true
    b. false

14. Actively participating in decisions regarding breast cancer treatment only makes a woman more anxious during the experience.
    a. true
    b. false

15. Seeking information about breast cancer from a variety of sources will help in making informed decisions.
    a. true
    b. false

Recovering From Surgery

T his chapter provides information on recovering from surgery.
We'll talk about ways to promote both physical and emotional health in women and their partners as they try to sta-
bilize their lives and achieve wellbeing.

NELLIE: *I was told by the doctors I would have a scar on my
breast, but then it wouldn't be anything visible when it
healed. But then they had to take the lymph nodes when
I had the lumpectomy.*

CAROL: *Right after surgery you have the discomfort, the scar,
things you can't do, you're restricted. . . . The worst part
for me was the mental part. Physical part, that wasn't
difficult. . . . It was just the nervousness; the fear was
the worst part for me*

GEORGE: *After the operation was over, Carol came up on the
stretcher and was in bed, I felt that at that point everything would work out. I felt that she was very strong.
Maybe she didn't realize how strong she was at the moment
but I thought she was very, very much in control.*

LINDA: *I was incredibly relieved. I so just wanted to live and get
rid of this cancer and I wasn't thinking about the cos-
metic things at that point. But I think later you do think
about that.*

The New York University (NYU) study on which this book is
based looked at the experience of women and their partners
throughout the first year after diagnosis and treatment of breast

cancer. Through our findings, we have identified the unique needs of women as they recover from surgery and the special needs of their partners, as well. They appear in Table 2.1

RECOGNIZE FEELINGS AFTER SURGERY

Women feel a great sense of relief when their breast cancer surgery is over. Their energy is now free to focus on physical healing. Since a hospital stay may be as brief as 1 day and seldom longer than 5 days, it is an important time to learn about recovery.

> LINDA: *As the week went on and I started to feel better and wasn't focusing on the pain that I was in and that type of thing, then I was anxious for what prognosis I was going to get about my nodes because that is the next thing that you're waiting to hear about. Were they positive, negative? How much, how many? Because, you know, you want to know whether it's metastasized further.*

Although a woman may have had fears about anesthesia and surgery, those fears may be replaced with concerns about surviving the disease itself.

How each partner deals with the findings of surgery may depend on personality factors, as well as adjustment to previous losses or disappointments in life. Even when the pathology report provides good news that the cancer is localized and not spread to the lymph nodes, some partners experience distress because they focus on what they see as the unpredictability of the future. A woman may question her choice of surgery and hope the right decision was made. Her partner, on the other hand, worries about his wife's adjustment to cancer, family finances, time off for doctor visits, and managing the household. When faced with the challenge of breast cancer, however, many couples become more aware of their own resources and experience a renewed inner strength.

PROMOTING PHYSICAL HEALING

Assessments by physicians and nurses are crucial to the early healing process. After surgery, the body gradually returns to normal.

TABLE 2.1   Needs of Women and Their Partners After Surgery

- Recognize feelings after surgery
- Identify ways to promote physical healing
- Develop strategies to adjust emotionally
- Create a support system
- Manage family and social roles

Nurses monitor blood pressure, pulse, breathing, and temperature as this process begins.

The first day after surgery, a bandage covers the incision site. It needs to be checked for any signs of bleeding or drainage. After surgery, a small drainage tube is usually placed in the surgical site. It is attached to a small container. Gentle suction is applied so that fluid does not accumulate under the skin. This helps the area to heal. Within a few days after surgery, the drainage usually subsides, and the tube is removed. The surgical site should be checked for any signs of infection such as redness, swelling, or warmth.

Most women and their partners are concerned about what the incision will look like. Some couples say it took courage to look at the incision for the first time, and they preferred to have their doctor or nurse with them. Linda's doctor helped her through the process.

LINDA: *He made it very obvious that he felt he had gotten good results and he had me see it very quickly. I thought it would be like, I don't know, days or something before they could remove the bandages. I think it was the next day that he said, "Now, I'm going to show you the wonderful results, your, you know, your new breast" and that type of thing. And he took the bandages down and made it something that was just very normal for me to see.*

NELLIE: *I was afraid of lymphedema, and I was told they wouldn't have to take a lot because the cancer was small, but they had to take a sample of the lymph nodes.*

If a total mastectomy or a modified radical mastectomy has been performed, then the breast has been removed. The incision is usually a thin, neat line that extends from the armpit across the chest toward the breast bone. The line is where the flaps of skin are brought together, or sutured, by either thread-like material or metal clips that look like staples. All incisions are red during the early healing process, but gradually fade over time.

Promoting Comfort, Reducing Pain

Comfort following surgery is important. Nurses will help the woman find a comfortable position either on her back or on the nonsurgical side, with the arm on the side of the surgery supported by a pillow. When sitting up, the arm on the affected side also should be supported by a pillow. This will promote good circulation and reduce arm swelling, called lymphedema. With today's surgical techniques, the incidence of arm swelling is greatly reduced.

It's very important to report pain to the nurse before it becomes too strong. The nurse will examine the dressing or drain. If the drain is not working well, there can be swelling under the skin that may cause pain. When pain medication is administered, it's wise to ask the nurse about the name and action of the medication, the dosage, and any potential side effects. With this information, one can better judge the effectiveness and any reactions one has to the medication.

LINDA: *You know, I've had surgeries in the past so I think I was used to how you feel after a surgery. For a woman who's never, ever had any kind of surgery, I think they will react a little more to the pain.*

Reconstruction immediately following breast surgery poses additional discomfort.

LINDA: *I think one of the things that was the worst, it wasn't so much the pain, there was pain there but it wasn't so much the pain. It was how different my body felt because he did a really good tummy tuck on me and so my skin had been pulled in very, very tight, and I kind of felt like somebody had cut out that nice middle elastic blubbery middle part of me and now I had a piece of board in there. It just felt so stiff and that was more, I think, odd saying, "Uh-oh, my body doesn't feel like me. How long will this last?"*

As an alternative to pain medication, or in addition to it, other ways to reduce discomfort may be considered that can include partners. Often a gentle back rub lessens discomfort and anxiety. The use of relaxation techniques and guided imagery also may increase a sense of well-being and lessen fatigue. Although comparing one's recovery process to someone else's is often a source of reassurance, it is important to realize that healing is an individual process.

Self-Care Activities

Promoting movement and circulation in the affected arm and shoulder is essential. Gently using the affected arm to eat, comb hair, or for other everyday activities will increase the range of motion.

The sooner a woman exercises her hand and arm muscles, she will be able to prevent stiffness and weakness in the muscles. She can start exercises that don't place stress on the incision almost immediately after surgery. She can squeeze a soft, round object such as a ball or orange. It is also important to bend and extend the fingers, wrist, and elbows at least three to five times a day, but not beyond the point of discomfort.

Within a day or 2 after surgery, walking is encouraged. The affected arm should be allowed to hang at the side first, then bent inward while walking.

It's not unusual to experience unusual or painful sensations in the breast following a mastectomy. These feelings may include mild pain, burning, or itching. They are normal and will go away gradually.

It's important to avoid injury and infection in the operative arm. The following care should be taken both in the hospital and at home.

- *Avoid medical procedures on affected arm.* Avoid taking blood pressures, drawing blood, or receiving injections in the affected arm.
- *Avoid injuries that may lead to infection.* Avoid burns, scratches, or other injury that may lead to infection in the affected arm and hand.
- *Cleanse any wounds promptly.* If an injury does occur, prompt cleansing of the wound is necessary to minimize the chance of infection.
- *Examine incision daily.* Examine the incision daily for signs of infection and report any redness, warmth, swelling, or discharge from the surgical site to the surgeon.

- *Pat incision dry.* A daily bath or shower is important to keep the skin clean once the incision is healed and the drain is removed. Following the shower, the incision should be patted dry.
- *Place sterile pad over incision.* A soft, sterile pad may be placed over the incision to prevent clothing from rubbing the skin.
- *Avoid deodorant and shaving under affected arm or creams on incision*

STRATEGIES TO PROMOTE PSYCHOLOGICAL RECOVERY

Just as physical healing takes time, so too does emotional healing. Grieving the temporary loss of health, or loss of a breast, will bring moments of denial, anger, or depression to both partners. In any one day, the gamut of these feelings may be experienced.

One way to help resolve the grief process may be to keep a journal. Writing down feelings and perceptions involves a process of connecting the inner and outer feelings. It serves as an outlet for emotions. As a journal is reviewed, partners may want to share their feelings and talk about their progress. One may experience a shift in perspective from fighting the enemy of illness to learning more about oneself.

> CAROL: *Every day I would write about my feelings and about just how I felt physically and it was just . . . very painful at times.*

Develop Strategies to Promote Emotional Healing

In the NYU study, it was found that one's sense of physical self is an integral part of one's emotional well being. And each woman is individual in how she feels about and responds to the profound physical changes that follow breast cancer surgery. Breast reconstruction raises as many different responses.

> LINDA: *I very consciously opted for it. I think it helped me psychologically. I think there is a grieving process for the fact that your old, familiar breast isn't there and it's gone. And, let's face it, I mean, with your sexuality, with feeling in*

> *that breast, it isn't the same. What I didn't have to go*
> *through, though, was having my body look so different,*
> *having to look at that loss and be reminded of it every day.*
> *Umm, I could forget. I didn't have to go through any*
> *prosthetic device issues. Bra shopping, I mean, I could still*
> *go for my old, familiar brand. So I think all those things*
> *helped. . . . Actually, in the plastic surgery end of it I*
> *think it's very important to do your homework and make*
> *sure, especially if you're having simultaneous reconstruc-*
> *tion, that your two doctors are working as a team.*

Whether choosing reconstruction or a prosthesis, it helps for a woman to communicate with her partner about her choice. For some men, it's not a big deal. For others, it is a big deal.

It is not unusual for women and their partners to have an adjustment period in reestablishing their sexual relationship. Difficulties may arise in either partner's sexual feelings. It is very important for each to be able to tell the other what is needed to have enjoyable and comfortable sex. For many couples, it is important to plan ahead so that there is time to create a relaxed and private atmosphere.

Women also may be concerned that if they are not interested in sex, they may be depriving their partner of sexual gratification. There may be times when having sex is not a priority, yet it is still important to maintain intimacy. Spending time together quietly, caressing, engaging in mutually enjoyable activities, and listening attentively, can be unifying and restoring.

Kathleen Conway, MSN, RN, CS, Clinical Director of the Center for Hope, advises, "If sex is important, they can still have sex. . . . Windows of opportunity (can be built in) between chemos, radiation, when there is energy. . . . If that was important before, it's going to be very important now. If it wasn't important before, it may be important now. And if it's not sexual, even the physical touching, holding, and the being close may be a priority. It's incredibly important for us as human beings and particularly when we're healing from an illness."

LINDA: *I think for me, Bob, first of all Bob was so supportive. I*
            never felt I was going to be any less because my breast
            was different. I think it was more of feeling sensations and
            things of that nature were very different.

BOB: *I know very strongly what Linda's breasts mean to her, her sexuality, and how hard that was. When she felt well enough to make love again, it was difficult. It was difficult for her, not for me. I was amazed. It really didn't change my feelings at all but I could see how it hurt her, how different it was for her own feeling and it was, again, I'm not patting myself on the back but I had to, I had to be super patient with the time it would take her to get used to her own body. And it took a long time and it's still going on but like she says, I'm amazed at how much she feels.*

Create a Support System

A woman receives support from many sources, including from her partner, who often feels a need to protect her. This support may sometimes feel controlling to a woman. In this case, partners or other family members or friend may have to change their behavior when they lend support.

GEORGE: *It was very difficult for me. I found that it was hard for me to really understand what Carol was going through. It was difficult for me to really feel what she was feeling.*

Family members are frequently the greatest source of both emotional and physical support. Yet they may experience their own distress and feel helpless or frustrated by not being able to relieve their loved one's pain. They, too, need an outlet for their stress or a shoulder to lean on. The challenge for a family is to achieve a balance between not enough focus on feelings as opposed to excessive concern.

Children also form their own perceptions when a parent becomes ill and exhibit their concerns in a number of ways. They may not want to leave their mother or may have difficulty focusing on their own activities and responsibilities. The natural tendency of parents is to protect a child from illness and often from a diagnosis of cancer. Yet, children are quite perceptive and realize that upsetting events are occurring.

LINDA: *We've been very, very open with the children. I mean, you know two of our children are adopted and we've*

> *always been very, very open about that issue. And this was no different. I mean, they were in the midst of this when this all happened.*

BOB: *I really don't believe, and Linda doesn't either, in hiding any of this from the kids because they know exactly what happened and in their own way as they grow, unless they're confronted with the fact that you can talk about these things and express yourself, cry about them, fear them, whatever, unless you can really do that it's only going to manifest itself some other way. So I always made sure we talked about it.*

In some cases, counseling may be beneficial. A renewed recognition of the importance of family relationships can encourage closeness and a greater appreciation of priorities in life.

Barbara Rabinowitz, Director of Oncology Services, Meridian Health Services, observes that "People will withdraw at times, sometimes because they feel overwhelmed by the feelings they have about the person who's going through the breast cancer experience. Sometimes they withdraw because of the fear of increasing the intimacy in the relationship because they mythologize perhaps that the diagnosis means that they will certainly lose that person and so they begin to protect themselves by withdrawing. Also people very often withdraw because they just don't know what to say. They don't realize that what they say is less important than their ability to listen."

In the process of recovery, enjoyable family activities can be planned as time and energy permit. An enjoyable occasion helps to recapture the "normal" times. It is a welcome diversion from the focus on the events associated with the treatment of the illness. Family members can also provide physical help to make these times possible. Help with laundry, cleaning, or shopping can be exactly the tangible aid that is needed to reduce pressures on the immediate family and give them more free time.

It is important to establish a supportive, trusting relationship with one's health care team. Women and their partners seek experts who will provide the best possible care and help them through this experience. They want help in making decisions about treatment, in coping with feelings about cancer as a life-threatening illness, and in dealing with their work and family responsibilities.

In the experience of Dr. Roy Ashikari, Vice President for Program Development, St. Agnes Hospital, White Plains, NY, "The trust between patient and the physician is the most important. . . . If the patient has a husband or boyfriend . . . we discuss this before surgery or before treatment. I think this is very, very important and this is not just a surgery. Once we do surgery we must follow this patient forever. We start right. Then . . . the patient trusts me and I trust the patient."

CAROL: *Well, I just felt that I totally relied on my doctor. I totally trusted him. I felt confident.*

LINDA: *I think women need to say there are some answers out there. Umm and it's not easy to pursue them, but don't give up. There are more there now than there had been when I first started, and it's an involving process and it's really helped us.*

BOB: *. . . Because if you're just a victim, you're going to be a victim of it and psychologically it takes over. It really helped us to know that, hey, we can do something here to help ourselves, to make it easier to get through this because even if it's just that we need another day, and if we ask for this and maybe we can work around this date.*

For some patients, a certain level of denial may help them to cope until they have the emotional strength and readiness to accept the diagnosis and treatment. In general, however, the open discussion of information with physicians, often reinforced by the nurse, and the inclusion of a partner or significant other, have been found to be helpful in absorbing information and ultimately adjusting to this experience.

Emotional healing from surgery is an ongoing process. Right after surgery, women and their partners talk about what they describe as an emotional roller coaster.

Barbara Rabinowitz finds that "What women say about their thoughts about survival and mortality when they've had a diagnosis of breast cancer is variable in that it changes along the process—where they are in the process from that first time that they hear a diagnosis of breast cancer to the time when they may be ending chemotherapy." There are a variety of experiences that people can have with depression, and it's not always easily recognized. People can experience listlessness, feeling disconnected from others, sleeplessness, loss of appetite. There are a variety of ways that the person can physically feel the reaction to depression in addition to the very understandable sadness that one might feel while going through the adaptations and adjustments.

> LINDA: *You know, I was 39 years old. I was dealing with my mortality. I was dealing with having a very young family. I was dealing with family issues of support that I thought I was going to get that I didn't; that I had to face up to because this was going to be another reality of life. And we were dealing with the stressors that we knew were going to be on our marriage during this period of time. Plus just the fact that my body wasn't the same anymore either.*

If feelings of depression or anxiety continue long after physical recovery, medical advice on counseling may be sought. The role of a partner in this healing process is important.

> LINDA: *I think you felt a little bit alone sometimes, though, because so much of the burden of the children was on you and I have to tell you, I mean, there was, in some ways I had to ask for help because, after you have the tramflap one of the things you can't do is lift for 6 weeks because of the possibility of a hernia. . . . And one thing that I did was I learned how to ask for some help instead of waiting for people to ask me. I think that's important. You know, when people say, "What do you need?" I think sometimes they need to focus on if there is a partner or significant other that's in the area, or somebody who can offer them the help.*

Community Resources

There are invaluable community resources that can help women as they create their external support system. The Reach to Recovery program of the American Cancer Society provides a hospital visit to women who have had surgery for breast cancer. Volunteers from the program have experienced breast cancer themselves and provide written materials on various topics.

They can provide patients with a soft, temporary breast form that may be worn when leaving the hospital. Within 6 to 8 weeks after surgery, a permanent breast prosthesis can be fitted when the swelling is gone and the surgical area is completely healed.

Information about breast prostheses is also available in department stores, medical supply stores, and specialty shops. It is important, however, to select an experienced provider. Most insurance companies will cover the cost of a breast prosthesis if it is approved by the physician.

MANAGING CHANGES IN FAMILY AND SOCIAL ROLES

The length of time needed to recover from breast cancer is often related to age, stage of the cancer, extent of surgery, and perhaps other things going on in each partner's life.

Within 4 to 6 weeks after surgery, most women have regained the motion in their arm to perform normal activities, yet some discomfort may be present for up to 3 months after surgery. Women who do not require any further treatment, such as chemotherapy or radiation, usually regain their original strength within 6 months.

After discharge from the hospital, the burden of office and hospital visits can be reduced if visits are scheduled at a time of day when energy levels are highest. Seek out staff in medical offices who can assist with information and directions to resources that are important in follow-up care. Anxiety about finding good follow-up care, or even going to a hospital or office for radiation or chemotherapy, is not uncommon.

It's important to focus on recovery, realizing that many challenges have already been successfully met. A close family member or friend may be helpful on these visits. Since the length of time in an office may be unpredictable initially, it may be less stressful to plan for a free half-day that permits an enjoyable outing after the visit. See Table 2.2 for tips on follow-up therapy.

The diagnosis and surgical treatment of breast cancer are significant stressors to both partners. It becomes important to delegate roles to avoid common stressors such as fatigue. For many women, an unexpected outcome of surgery is significantly less energy.

TABLE 2.2   Tips on Follow-Up Therapy

- Plan visits for when energy level is highest
- Use staff as an information resource
- Focus on recovery
- Bring a family member or friend
- Schedule an outing after visit
- Identify questions to be asked of the physician or nurse

"Fatigue can surface and resurface along the continuum from diagnosis through treatment on to adjuvant therapy and then to rehabilitation," states Barbara Rabinowitz. "It is a big piece of what women complain about, both with chemotherapy and with radiation therapy. A really draining kind of fatigue. Happily, it most often resolves when the treatment is done or soon thereafter, but it's hard for people to endure while they're going through it."

During this time of physical and psychological healing, it's important to achieve a balance between activities and frequent periods of rest. Sometimes this means spreading out home or work-related responsibilities throughout the course of the day, or doing them in ways that conserve energy. Recognizing and following body rhythms is essential to regaining a sense of well-being. And a partner may experience similar symptoms due to distress over the situation and assuming more responsibilities in the home and elsewhere.

Both partners need to be patient with themselves and understand that adjustment takes time. They need to learn to request support from family or friends and let go of certain responsibilities. This will reduce both the physical and emotional load and the level of fatigue.

Self-Care

Care at home in other ways is important in regaining and maintaining health.

A diet with proteins and vitamins promotes healing in the surgical area. Although information on a low-fat diet and risk of breast cancer is conflicting, many breast cancer specialists believe that less than 20% fat is beneficial. The American Cancer Society suggests reducing total fat, eating high-fiber foods such as whole grain cereals, fruits and vegetables, and including foods rich in vitamins A and C. Lowering the amount of fat may alter the metabolism of certain hormones and decrease the risk of cancer. Some studies suggest that alcohol may increase the risk of breast cancer, so limited use is recommended.

Finally, comfort and safety are important. Wearing a seat belt is important for protection but a shoulder strap may be irritating to the incision. This can be alleviated by placing a soft pillow or blanket between the chest and the seat belt. A breast prosthesis may actually provide additional protection and comfort.

SUMMARY

We hope this chapter provides many of the tools needed to recognize the value of feelings after surgery, identify ways to promote physical healing, develop strategies to adjust emotionally, create a support system, and manage family and social roles. Most of all, it is important to focus on a positive attitude, the priorities of one's life, and complete recovery.

KNOWLEDGE REVIEW:
RECOVERING FROM SURGERY

Content Outline

This section includes an outline of the content of the chapter. It may be used as a review of the key points, or as a helpful aide to health professionals in preparing educational materials for patients.

I. Feelings after surgery
   A. Common feelings and concerns
      1. sense of relief
      2. concerns about surviving
      3. unpredictable future
      4. question choices and decisions
      5. family finances
      6. loss of time from work
      7. managing the household
      8. renewed inner strength
II. Physical recovery
   A. Assessment by physicians and nurses
      1. blood pressure
      2. pulse
      3. breathing
      4. temperature
      5. check bandage for bleeding and drainage
      6. drainage tube with gentle suction
      7. signs of infection
         a. redness
         b. swelling
         c. warmth
   B. Appearance of incision
      1. concerns about what it will look like
      2. lumpectomy incision
         a. usually a few inches long
         b. second incision in underarm if lymph nodes removed
      3. mastectomy incision
         a. thin line extending from armpit across the chest toward the breast bone
      4. all incisions red during healing, fade over time

    C. Promoting comfort, reducing pain
        1. positioning
        2. reporting pain
        3. asking about pain medication
        4. alternative methods to reduce pain
           a. back rub
           b. relaxation
           c. guided imagery
        5. promoting movement and circulation
        6. walking
        7. recognizing phantom sensations
    D. Avoid injury and infection in operative arm
        1. avoid medical procedures on affected arm
        2. avoid burns, scratches, that can lead to infection
        3. cleanse any wounds promptly
        4. examine incision daily
        5. keep skin clean: wash and pat dry
        6. cover incision with sterile pad to prevent clothing from rubbing
        7. avoid deodorants and creams
III. Emotional healing
    A. Grieving for loss of health or loss of breast
        1. denial
        2. anger
        3. depression
    B. Strategies to promote emotional healing
        1. keep a journal
        2. share feelings about surgery, body image, and sexuality.
        3. communicate feelings about reconstruction
        4. plan for reestablishing sexual relationship
           a. changes in interest
           b. explore alternate ways of expressing intimacy
    C. Emotional recovery an ongoing process
        1. described as an emotional roller coaster
        2. need to recognize depression
IV. Create an effective support system
    A. Common sources of support
        1. partner
        2. other family members
        3. children

    B. Recognize family members often experience distress too

    C. Consider counselling

    D. Plan family activities

    E. Accept help with household tasks

    F. Establish supportive, trusting relationships with health care team

    G. Explore community resources

        1. Reach to Recovery

        2. American Cancer Society

V. Manage changes in family and social roles

    A. Recovery at home

    B. Office and hospital visits

        1. plan when energy level is highest

        2. use staff as information resource

    C. Follow up therapy

        1. focus on recovery

        2. bring a family member or friend

        3. schedule on outing after visit

    D. Avoid fatigue

        1. delegating roles

        2. spread out home and work related responsibilities throughout the course of the day

        3. recognize and follow body rhythms

        4. request and accept help from friends

    E. Take care of self

        1. diet

        2. comfort and safety

Test Your Knowledge: Study Questions

Directions: Circle the letter corresponding to the correct response in each of the following.

1. Following breast surgery it is uncommon to wonder whether the correct surgical choice was made.
   a. true
   b. false

2. You can expect the nurse to frequently check temperature, pulse, blood pressure and bandage right after surgery
   a. true
   b. false

3. In rare situations women may have a tube in place that drains fluid from the incision following surgery.
   a. true
   b. false

4. Redness and swelling of the incision along with a slight fever after breast surgery should be reported to the health care provider.
   a. true
   b. false

5. Most women are comfortable looking at their surgical site soon after mastectomy.
   a. true
   b. false

6. The best time to ask for pain medication following surgery is before the pain becomes too intense.
   a. true
   b. false

7. Exercising the arm and shoulder soon after breast surgery is recommended.
   a. true
   b. false

8. Bathing or showering is not permitted until the breast incision is completely healed.
   a. true
   b. false

9. It is unusual for a woman to feel a sense of grieving during the postoperative recovery phase.
    a. true
    b. false

10. Women are encouraged to express feelings of sadness after breast surgery.
    a. true
    b. false

11. It is suggested that family members keep breast cancer related fears and concerns to themselves.
    a. true
    b. false

12. Many describe the experience of breast cancer as "a smooth gradual process of recovery."
    a. true
    b. false

13. If a woman frequently feels isolated and depressed following breast surgery, she should recognize that these feelings are expected and they will pass.
    a. true
    b. false

14. Following surgery for breast cancer friends and family members often know how to provide support, but they are reluctant to do so.
    a. true
    b. false

15. Family roles and responsibilities need to change during the first few months following breast surgery.
    a. true
    b. false

3

Understanding Adjuvant Therapy

Adjuvant therapy refers to the treatments given in addition to surgical treatment of breast cancer. Chemotherapy, radiation, and hormone therapy are all types of adjuvant therapies.

The goals of this chapter are to describe the kinds of adjuvant therapies and indications for each, to consider factors related to decision making, and to identify resources to guide women in making decisions about adjuvant therapy. We'll provide information on enhancing physical and emotional health during treatment; promoting and accepting support from family and community resources; and learning how to set realistic personal goals during treatment.

LINDA: *I remember a doctor in Boston saying to me, "What do you think the worst things about chemotherapy are going to be for you? Or the biggest symptomology that you're going to have?" And of course the first thing that comes to your mind is, oh, you know, nausea. You know, I'm going to be throwing up and all of this type of thing and losing my hair and that type of thing. And I remember him saying to me, "No." He said, "It's going to be fatigue and not weight loss but weight gain with breast cancer protocols."*

CAROL: *I was very afraid of the radiation but I was afraid not to have it, I was afraid to have it. My two girlfriends, they each had mastectomies because they went before me, but they didn't have radiation so not only was the cancer a fear, the radiation was a fear for me.*

47

TYPES OF ADJUVANT THERAPIES
AND INDICATIONS

First, we'll describe the kinds of adjuvant therapies available, and the indications for each one. Adjuvant therapy is the treatment administered to minimize the risk of a future cancer recurrence.

Adjuvant *systemic* therapy refers to a drug or substance that is spread by way of the blood stream throughout the body. This includes chemotherapy and hormone therapy.

Adjuvant therapy that is *localized,* on the other hand, refers to radiation treatments to a limited part of the body. Radiation treatment is the recommended treatment following a breast-conserving surgery, such as lumpectomy. It is administered directly to the breast to destroy any cancer cells that may remain. It is also sometimes administered to the lymph nodes under the axilla.

Chemotherapy

Chemotherapy refers to anticancer drugs that destroy rapidly dividing cancer cells (Figure 3.1) that have travelled into the lymph system or blood stream from the primary tumor (Figure 3.2). Chemotherapy drugs are given in a number of different ways. Some may be given in the form of a pill, some like a flu shot, and others are given directly into the vein.

> LINDA: *I think when it came to the chemotherapy it was a little bit different. I was very lucky to have my nodes negative so there were actually a lot of options out there for me. . . . I took all my test results, which were all numbers to me, and I staged my cancer so that before I went to the oncologist I kind of knew, based on size, type of cells, and that kind of thing, where I was with my cancer and what stage it was at. And from there I went for three opinions.*

There are numerous factors that an oncologist considers in advising a patient on what kinds of adjuvant therapy should be considered. Following surgery, the laboratory report will provide information based on the microscopic examination of the tumor that has been removed. This information is crucial to making decisions about adjuvant therapy. One important factor is whether any cancer cells were found in the lymph nodes. If more than one

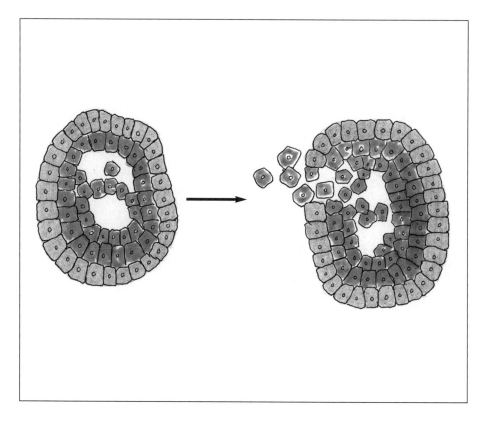

FIGURE 3.1 Illustration of rapidly dividing cancer cells.

lymph node was removed, the report will indicate how many nodes contained cancer cells. Positive node status means that cancer cells are present. A second factor is whether the tumor tends to "attract" or "bind" with estrogen. Tumors are either positive or negative in terms of estrogen receptor status. A third factor is the size of the tumor. A fourth factor is the rate of growth of the tumor cells, known as the S-phase fraction. A tumor that divides rapidly is known to have a high S-phase fraction. Information on the type of cancer cells, specific growth factors, and the nuclear grade of the tumor is an important part of the pathology report. Table 3.1 lists the factors that are assessed in considering adjuvant therapy. An oncologist also considers individual factors, such as age of the patient, menopausal status, and general health.

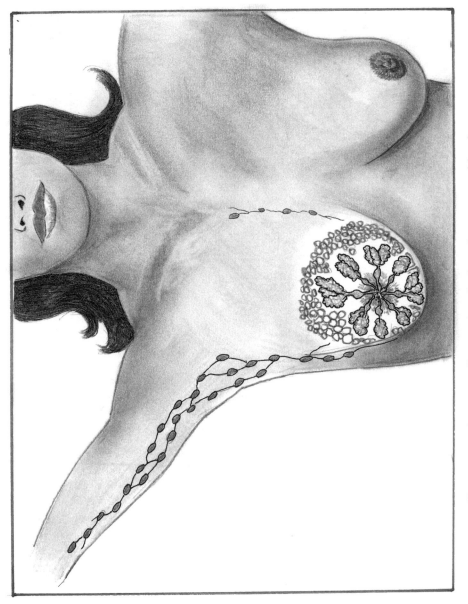

FIGURE 3.2 Illustration of cancer cells entering the lymph system or blood stream.

TABLE 3.1   Factors Related to Adjuvant Therapy

- Negative nodes—no cancer cells
- Positive nodes—cancer cells present
- Estrogen receptor status—tumor tends to "attract" or "bind" with estrogen
- Size of tumor
- Rate of growth—high S-phase fraction: tumor divides rapidly
- Nuclear grade of tumor

Dr. Abraham Mittelman, an oncologist at New York Medical College and St. Agnes Hospital in White Plains, NY, describes his approach: "One has to look at the patient as a whole, not just the cancer, but also understand their other medical illnesses, the ability of this patient to tolerate chemotherapy, and obviously look at the risks and benefits that one would achieve from the chemotherapy. If you compare groups of women who got chemo versus groups of women who did not get chemo, it is clear that chemotherapy reduces the recurrence of breast cancer by 30%, and reduces death rate or mortality from breast cancer by about 25%."

Current thinking on adjuvant therapy is based on about 400 clinical trials, including more than 220,000 women (Hortobagyi, 1998). Hormonal therapy and chemotherapy added to local treatment, or radiation, appear to favorably alter the incidence of recurrence. Combination chemotherapy is more effective than single-drug therapy in reducing the annual risk of death. Although the effects of combination chemotherapy appear to be more marked in women younger than 60 years, especially those who are premenopausal when therapy is begun, the effectiveness has been clearly demonstrated up to the age of 69 years.

Chemotherapy is given intravenously or by mouth, depending on the drug. The drugs travel in the bloodstream throughout the entire body. The most common combinations of drugs (NCCN & ACS, 1999) are:

- cyclophosphamide, methotrexate, and fluorouracil (CMF);
- cyclophosphamide, doxorubicin (Adriamycin), and fluorouracil (CAF);
- doxorubicin (Adriamycin) and cyclophosphamide (AC), with or without paclitaxel (Taxol);
- doxorubicin (Adriamycin) followed by CMF

Hormone Therapy

Tamoxifen, a form of hormone therapy, is often recommended as another type of adjuvant therapy. Tamoxifen is an antiestrogen, meaning that it binds to an estrogen receptor. By blocking estrogen, it potentially reduces the stimulus that the estrogen offers to growth of cancer cells. Although there are other hormone therapies, they are all designed to have an anti-estrogen effect.

Tamoxifen is thought to hold considerable promise for prevention. The National Surgical Adjuvant Breast and Bowel Project (NSABP) indicated that in a study of over 13,000 healthy women at risk of breast cancer because of age (60 years or older), or younger women who were at increased risk because of a family history, age at menarche, nulliparity, or previous benign breast biopsy, a significant ($p < .00001$) 49% reduction in the incidence of breast cancer was noted. The women were randomized to receive tamoxifen 20 mg/day or placebo. After about 4 years of follow-up, this effect was considered to be sufficiently robust to stop the trial, unblind the randomization, and offer tamoxifen to all participants on placebo (Powles, 1999, p. 21).

Although studies have shown that tamoxifen significantly reduces the risks of recurrence and death in all age groups afflicted with breast cancer (Hortobagyi, 1998), the role of chemotherapy and tamoxifen among pre- and postmenopausal women is complicated. It used to be thought that premenopausal women would benefit from chemotherapy but not from tamoxifen, in contrast to postmenopausal women who were thought to benefit from tamoxifen but not from chemotherapy. However, the current thinking is that, depending on the factors presented in Table 3.2, both of these groups may benefit from chemotherapy and both may benefit from tamoxifen as well.

Dr. Abraham Mittelman describes the decision-making process as follows: "The question is when would you use tamoxifen? Clearly, in women who are estrogen-receptor positive, tamoxifen use is recommended, and it's been shown by a number of studies that tamoxifen reduces the recurrence of breast cancer in the contralateral, or other breast, by 50%. So it's an important agent to use. And it is also recommended that tamoxifen should be used for 5 years."

TABLE 3.2   Indiciations for Adjuvant Therapy

- Premenopausal women with positive nodes = chemotherapy
- Premenopausal women with negative nodes = possible chemotherapy or tamoxifen depending on size and characteristics of tumor
- Postmenopausal women with negative nodes = usually no chemotherapy
- Postmenopausal women with positive nodes = hormone therapy and/or chemotherapy
- Pre- and postmenopausal women = tamoxifen likely to reduce recurrence
- Lumpectomy patients = surgery with radiation, possibly other forms of adjuvant therapy

Radiation

If a woman has a lumpectomy, radiation is recommended as the primary adjuvant therapy. The reason for radiation therapy is because breast cancer can occur in the breast in different places at the same time. This may not show on a mammogram or be found by physical examination. The usual dose is 4500 to 5000 rads over 5 to 6 weeks. Treatments may include a final boost of 1000 rads at the site of original tumor. Radiation treatments should not be given if there have been prior radiation treatments to the breast, if the woman is pregnant, or if the woman has certain other diseases.

Side effects of radiation are most likely to become more evident as treatments progress. Common side effects include:

- Swelling and heaviness in the breast
- Sunburn-like skin changes in the treated area
- Skin sensitivity
- Fatigue

Changes to the breast tissue and skin usually disappear in 6 to 12 months. In some women, the breast becomes smaller and firmer after radiation therapy. Radiation of axillary lymph nodes can also cause lymphadema.

NELLIE: *You feel fatigued. It's very exhausting, especially if you have to travel. And you don't experience that until the*

> *third week, because it was a 6-week treatment. You start*
> *feeling fatigued, you know, after 3 weeks.*

CAROL: *The worst times were in the evening in bed. I had to get*
          a prescription to take something to calm me because I
          couldn't sleep at all. Everything came out at night and
          I was just panicky.

Pre- and postmenopausal women with positive nodes typically require adjuvant therapy. Doctors may recommend premenopausal women with negative nodes to have chemotherapy, primarily if the size or characteristics of the tumor warrant it. Postmenopausal women with negative nodes are generally not treated with chemotherapy. Tamoxifen is considered to be of benefit to both groups in reducing the chance of recurrence. Finally, lumpectomy patients usually have surgery with radiation. Some may have chemotherapy as well.

Remember that the decision to use adjuvant therapy should follow a thorough discussion between a woman, her partner, and her oncologist. They will want to consider the risks of the therapy, and the impact on quality of life.

GETTING MORE INFORMATION
ON TREATMENT

Now that you have an understanding of the types of adjuvant therapies and the indications for them, you may wonder how to find the right resources to guide you through the process. We'll explore those questions now.

Should a couple settle on one opinion? What should they ask of their potential oncologist? Following an initial consultation with an oncologist or radiologist, some couples wish to seek a second opinion on adjuvant therapy. They also will want to be certain whether their health insurance will be accepted as payment for services.

If the surgery was performed in a large medical center, someone at that institution may be consulted. Such a decision often allows the breast surgeon and the oncologist to work together in developing a treatment plan.

Adjuvant therapies are given by medical oncologists and radiation oncologists. A medical oncologist is a physician who evaluates the patient, determines the use of chemotherapy, and administers the chemotherapy. A radiation oncologist evaluates the patient to determine the amount of radiation that will be administered, the areas to which the radiation will be given, and the angles or the direction by which the radiation is going to be applied to minimize side effects of radiation.

BOB: *It was hard at that point. She got three completely different opinions, and it was really, I mean, at that point it was, "Okay, which one do we pick?" One was a very strong attack. One was in the middle. One was a lot less. So you have to choose.*

LINDA: *I think this is where the woman has to realize you've got to make your own decisions. In the beginning you just want somebody to take care of you and to tell you what to do. . . . Initially I went into this without having done a lot of research except all the pamphlets I was finding in the doctor's office, and I just was very lucky to have doctors who were educating me, who were pushing me to be educated.*

BOB: *I just didn't want to have her suffer more than she had to so I was leaning toward the least painful one that would work. But I really didn't force an opinion. Just told her whatever she wanted to do I had total faith in whatever she decided.*

LINDA: *I did decide to have the chemotherapy but I had more of a middle of the road protocol rather than the most aggressive one, and one of the cancer centers in Boston told me I could opt not to have any at all.*

Women and their partners should consider these questions for the oncologist:

- Who will administer the treatments?
- How long will each treatment last?
- What will the treatment feel like?

- In what kind of a setting will the treatments be given?
- Is blood work required during the course of treatment?
- Can the treatments be scheduled at times that are most convenient?
- What kind of side effects might occur?
- How can the side effects be controlled?

"I think a doctor who will listen is most important," explains Kathleen Conway, MSN, RN, CS, Clinical Director of the Center for Hope, who counsels breast cancer patients and their families. "A doctor who takes your questions seriously, who makes time for you, who's available, who doesn't mind when you go for a second opinion, in fact encourages you to do that, and is willing to talk to other doctors, maybe your internist, and keeps good communication going."

Getting answers to questions and knowing what to expect will make coping easier. And remember, side effects are limited in time.

While there can be temporary discomfort related to adjuvant therapy, many patients in the NYU study actually described a sense of emotional security from the protection the therapy offered.

Once one feels secure with one's oncologist and treatment plan, the journey through adjuvant therapy will be less stressful.

ENHANCING PHYSICAL AND EMOTIONAL HEALTH

A woman may experience discomfort from adjuvant therapy, but she will tolerate it better if the physical recovery from surgery is smooth and uncomplicated. It's especially important to promote the healing process. Focusing on emotional well-being is an important part of the process.

It is natural to have concerns about adjuvant therapy, including potential side effects, because we all tend to fear the unknown. The more information a woman has, the less anxiety she will feel about the treatments. Also, completion of a first treatment reduces fears of the unknown, and starts one off on a plan for managing one's own care.

LINDA: *I think what kept me going was I desperately wanted to live. I had had a baby after 15 years of infertility in the same year I got the cancer. I had two adopted, beautiful boys that I wanted to live for who had already gone through a loss in their life. . . . And I think we both agreed on that attitude early on after the initial shock wore off and I just wasn't going to give in.*

Managing Side Effects

In general, chemotherapy involves the use of strong drugs that attack any rapidly dividing cancer cells. The cells of the stomach, intestines, skin in the mouth, hair, and bone marrow may also be affected because they contain rapidly dividing cells.

As a result of the effects on the stomach and intestines, there may be nausea in the first days following a treatment. New antinausea medications can help control this uncomfortable side effect. Mouth sores also may develop. The discomforts can be modified by a baking soda mouthwash and the avoidance of spicy foods.

LINDA: *I took my chemotherapy in the middle of the week knowing that that's when I was going to have my reaction and that's when I was going to feel both the worse for me from a fatigue standpoint and also a nausea standpoint.*

Hair loss is another dismaying side effect of chemotherapy. Hair loss may involve not only scalp hair but eyebrows, lashes, pubic, and other body hair. Women may want to buy a wig before hair loss occurs. If hair thinning or loss occurs, it is important to remember that it is temporary—it will grow back. Many of the women in the NYU study chose to wear wigs, or scarves, or interesting hats, when going out. Attention to makeup and attractive new outfits also helps to enhance self-image and helps one feel attractive. The Look Good, Feel Better program, located throughout the country, helps women enhance their self-image during adjuvant therapy.

LINDA: *I went to try on wigs and maybe it was because of the color. Nobody had my color and I was trying on these white wigs and these black wigs and I was looking kind of hysterical, and we were laughing about it. And I decided I was going to go with scarves, turbans. I'm a hat person, so that appealed to me. But I was lucky. Fifty percent of the people on the type of protocol that I was on do not lose their hair so I lost only about a third of my hair. It was kind of see-through, and I remember the kids saying, "Oh, wow, Mommy, you know, do you know that you really hardly have any eyelashes?" So I went out and I got, you know, the big clump mascara, you know, the kind that lengthens and thickens and I wore that every day.*

Radiation

Radiation's side effects are generally less intense than chemotherapy and are related to the radiation technique, the dose, and the total radiation given. Side effects may include fatigue, reddening of the skin, minor changes in skin texture, and sensitivity. Occasionally the patient may develop some radiation effect on the lungs because they are right behind the breast.

Tamoxifen

Because tamoxifen is an antiestrogen drug, its side effects may be similar to those of menopause. They may include mood swings, fluid retention, nausea, hot flashes, and a decrease in white blood cells and platelets. Tamoxifen may also increase the risk for uterine cancer.

Women taking tamoxifen should be monitored by a gynecologist and should have an ultrasound examination of the uterus once or twice a year for 5 years.

AVOID INFECTIONS OR ILLNESS—REPORT ANY SIGNS TO DOCTOR

The white cells and platelets may be lowered as a result of chemotherapy and this, in turn, reduces resistance to colds or flu. It is important to avoid infections. If signs of an infection or other illness occur, such as fever or pain, they should be reported to the physician.

MAINTAIN GOOD NUTRITION

It is vital to maintain good nutrition during chemotherapy. The first part of a good nutrition plan is a well-balanced diet. It is helpful to select favorite fruits and vegetables and eat them as snacks between meals. Bland foods may be tolerated better. In addition, fat in the diet should be decreased by limiting butter and eating leaner meats like chicken and fish. Drinking less fluids with meals may also improve nausea.

> BOB: . . . *Nutritionally, we've not made any big changes. We always eat a lot of vegetables and fruit and a lot of home cooking and, you know, we weren't junk food junkies and all of a sudden realized we can't do that. What we wanted to change was to get a little more exercise, but we haven't done that.*

> CAROL: *Basically, overall lots of fruits and salads and healthy foods. I think it's important, and it makes me feel that I'm doing the right thing.*

A frequently discussed side effect of chemotherapy or hormone therapy is weight gain. Although the cause of weight gain is unclear, it is believed to be related to a change in metabolism, rather than to a change in dietary habits. Adequate nutrition is very important to the healing process. Weight reduction through serious dieting is not recommended. A sensible goal is to return to a comfortable weight after therapy is completed. Because weight gain at this time can be upsetting, a woman might want to consider treating herself to a new outfit or two that makes her feel both comfortable and attractive.

> Linda: *I had a tendency to sit down after dinner and be somewhat inactive because I was beat by the end of the day. And I think that's where some of the weight gain comes in; because you're used to being much more active.*

PLAN FREQUENT PERIODS OF REST WITH A BALANCE OF ACTIVITY

Fatigue, a burdensome side effect, is often associated with chemotherapy, as well. Depending on the particular drug, fatigue may be related to suppression of the bone marrow, which decreases the blood count. Planning frequent periods of rest while maintaining a balance of activity is helpful.

LINDA: *The fatigue was really difficult. Because of the fact that I had young children I couldn't just come home from work then and just lie down. But the nausea was not as bad. I think there are things that can be given to you now, and as long as you're making sure that you're doing what your doctor has prescribed that was very helpful. I needed to have my time to sleep. I mean, I got into a regimen with that. Bob was really supportive of that. And I think the chemotherapy probably went better than we both expected. . . . I tried to plan around the fatigue and how I was going to feel, and one of the things that I did was I made sure it was okay at work, well, I actually went in and I told them at work that this is what I wanted.*

MANAGE MENOPAUSE-LIKE SYMPTOMS

Chemotherapy over a long period of time also may affect the menstrual cycle. In premenopausal women, chemotherapy can induce an early menopause, or the ability to conceive may be affected. Since the production of estrogen normally decreases in menopause, this may result in a reduced interest in sexual activities and vaginal dryness. Vaginal lubricants can be used to provide additional moisture and enhance comfort if needed.

LINDA: *I think what was more difficult was the fact that chemotherapy put me into menopause and that caused changes in sexuality that were kind of compounded by this, and that hit me all at once because it was a chemically induced menopause.*

BOB: *. . . I'm not an expert on technical, the medical technical end of it, but there's no vaginal secretions and there really was no relations. Very painful. . . . There's a lot of patience involved.*

OTHER MANAGEMENT STRATEGIES

A soft, loose undergarment, as well as skin cream, will reduce any discomfort. Mild swelling in the arm and limitation of mobility are occasionally reported. Physical exercises of the arm during the treatment period are important and should keep swelling to a minimum.

Some couples in the NYU study marked off the dates on a calendar as each treatment was completed. They became very resourceful in finding ways to manage the treatments and their side effects while enjoying many other aspects of their lives.

Stress Management

It's well documented that inner peace and a stress-free quality of life promote healing. Many couples say that hope and spiritual wellbeing are very important in maintaining a positive outlook and providing the inner strength to face the difficult times. Some increase their spiritual wellbeing through prayer and meditation, while others seek support from their clergy or members of their church or synagogue.

NELLIE: *There was a church in my neighborhood that I made phone calls to, and I started going to Bible studies, you know, and they gave me some sections of the Bible. So I would read it and meditate on it. And that is what led me through this time, and continually, actually.*

Many people find that by exploring the meaning of illness, feelings of anger and depression have a better chance of being resolved.

CAROL: *I had difficulty with George, he was wonderful through the whole thing, but then when it was over, it was over, and let's get on with life. . . . I kept a diary and I needed to talk to people who had been through the same thing.*

George: *I really enjoy my work, and I'm out there every day. I mean, I have to give it everything to make it successful, I feel, and so that's what I do.*

LINDA: *And for me, when I'm really down, or I need a lift, a lot of times for me people will really help that so I continued to entertain and, you know, sometimes I mean, I was really tired from it, but that's the kind of thing that helped.*

BOB: *When we say entertain, we didn't have, you know, they weren't parties for just grown-ups. They were our family,*

> *our friends with their kids. . . . I also do a lot of music,*
> *so when I had a minute I would write, I did a lot of writ-*
> *ing during those years. . . . When I'm lonely or sad, I'm*
> *writing that way. It's a really saving grace for me.*

Many couples in the NYU study said that a sense of control is vital to a successful and healthy recovery. The choice to actively participate in the recovery process is consistent with what couples describe as their "fighting spirit" to conquer both the cancer and their fears.

Kathleen Conway explains, "What's most important is that the woman be in charge because she feels so out of control and so devastated with the initial diagnosis. When she can take control and take charge and feel that she is in a sense not at the mercy of the doctors but actually has control over that, who she sees."

Coping with the disruptive events related to surgery and adjuvant therapy is a significant challenge. How a woman and her partner deal with the challenges depends on their own inner strength, support from others, and even prior experience with persons living with cancer.

Sharing the experience with others can be beneficial, especially other breast cancer patients and their partners. Sometimes this is a friend, other times it may be women in a support group for the patient, and extended family for the partner. Sharing your feelings and concerns is a healthy way of coping.

BOB: *There's so much going on, so much caregiving between*
         what Linda needed, the food that had to be cooked, the
         kids had to be driven around and taken care of, the house
         chores, fixing the house, there's so much to do that
         there's not a lot of time to really give yourself what you
         think you need.

Often a crisis in our lives makes us reevaluate our priorities. It is an opportunity to get in touch with our inner selves and to connect intimately with those who share our lives. Times of crisis can also be times of growth. When the difficult challenges of adjuvant therapy are in the past, couples may actually see how much they have grown personally.

"I think a woman needs to come and talk," says Kathleen Conway, "I think it's helpful for her to talk with other women as well as perhaps to get counseling for herself and her husband." Sometimes another person who has been through cancer treatment can be a great source of support. There are cancer support groups who offer this kind of opportunity.

BOB: *I needed to talk to somebody who didn't, who didn't know me. I needed to get something off my chest.*

Set Realistic Personal Goals During Treatment

Many couples say that it is helpful to focus on the idea of living with breast cancer instead of possibly dying from cancer. Although difficult at times, following a usual routine can help to maintain a sense of normalcy. The important thing is to set realistic personal goals, particularly during treatment.

We hope that this chapter helps to establish a positive experience and a base of knowledge from which a woman and her partner may make the best choices and effectively cope with the physical and emotional challenges of breast cancer.

KNOWLEDGE REVIEW: ADJUVANT THERAPY

Content Outline

This section provides an outline of the content of the chapter. It may be used as a review of the key points, or as a helpful aid to health professionals in preparing educational materials for patients.

I. Kinds of adjuvant therapies and indications for use
   A. Systemic therapy
      1. treats whole body
      2. spread by way of blood system
         a. chemotherapy
         b. hormone therapy
   B. Localized therapy
      1. treats limited part of body
         a. radiation therapy
      2. recommended following lumpectomy
      3. used to destroy remaining cancer cells
   C. Chemotherapy actions
      1. destroy rapidly dividing cancer cells that have traveled into the lymph system or blood stream from primary tumor
      2. given by pill, shot, or into vein
   D. Factors influencing type of adjuvant therapy
      1. staging of disease
         a. size of tumor
         b. spread to lymph nodes or distant sites
         c. characteristics of tumor
      2. other factors
         a. age of patient
         b. estrogen/progesterone receptor sites
         c. other medical conditions
         d. menopausal status
         e. lifestyle factors
   E. Tamoxifen
      1. antiestrogen
      2. used in women who are estrogen receptor positive
      3. reduces recurrences
      4. one tablet in morning and at night
      5. recommended to be taken for five years

    F. Indications for radiation therapy
       1. used following breast conserving surgery
       2. typically given for five weeks on a daily basis
       3. contraindications for radiation
         a. prior radiation to breast
         b. pregnancy
         c. certain other diseases
II. Factors related to decision making
    A. Premenopausal women with positive nodes
       1. chemotherapy
    B. Premenopausal women with negative nodes
       1. possible chemotherapy
       2. Tamoxifen depending on size and characteristics of tumor
    C. Postmenopausal women with negative nodes
       1. usually no chemotherapy
    D. Postmenopausal women with positive nodes
       1. hormone therapy and/or chemotherapy
    E. Pre- and postmenopausal women
       1. Tamoxifen likely to reduce recurrence
       2. Possibly other forms of adjuvant therapy
    F. Lumpectomy patients
       1. radiation following surgery
III. Resources for guidance on decision making
    A. Types of oncologist
       1. medical oncologist
         a. evaluates the patient
         b. determines the use of chemotherapy
         c. administers the chemotherapy
       2. radiation oncologist
         a. evaluates the patient
         b. determines the amount of radiation patient receives
         c. determines the areas radiation is to be given
         d. determines angles or direction radiation is applied
    B. Choosing an oncologist
       1. chemistry between patient and physician
       2. seek second opinion
       3. investigate health insurance
IV. Enhancing physical and emotional health
    A. Concerns about potential side effects of chemotherapy
       1. affects rapidly dividing cells

        a. stomach
        b. intestines
        c. skin in mouth
        d. hair
        e. bone marrow
    2. common side effects of chemotherapy
        a. nausea
        b. mouth sores
        c. temporary hair loss
        d. reduced resistance to infection and colds
        e. weight gain
        f. fatigue
        g. early menopause
        h. changes in sexuality
    3. controlling side effects of chemotherapy
        a. antinausea medications
        b. baking soda mouthwash
        c. avoiding spicy foods
        d. use of wigs, scarves, and hats
        e. use of makeup to enhance self-image
        f. avoid infections
        g. exercise as tolerated
        h. maintain good nutrition
        i. plan frequent periods of rest
        j. use of vaginal lubricants if needed
  B. Side effects of tamoxifen
    1. mood swings
    2. hot flashes
    3. increased risk of uterine cancer
        a. need for regular gynecologist exam
  C. Managing side effects of radiation
    1. reddening of the skin
    2. minor changes in skin texture
    3. sensitivity
        a. soft loose fitting undergarments
        b. skin creams
    4. swelling of arm, limited mobility
        a. physical exercise of arm
  D. Questions for physicians
    1. Who will administer treatment?

       2. How long will each treatment last?
       3. What will treatment feel like?
       4. In what kind of setting will the treatment be given?
       5. Is blood work required during the course of treatment?
       6. Can the treatments be scheduled at times that are most convenient?
       7. What kind of side effects might occur?
       8. How can the side effects be controlled?
    E. Stress management
       1. maintain positive outlook
       2. maintain hope and spiritual well-being
          a. prayer and meditation
          b. support from clergy or church
          c. explore meaning of illness
       3. maintain sense of control
V. Promote and accept support
    A. Share experiences with others
    B. Accept help with household chores
    C. Reevaluate priorities
    D. Connect with others with similar experiences
       1. explore support groups
    E. Consider counselling
VI. Set realistic personal goals during treatment
    A. Focus on idea of living with breast cancer
    B. Follow usual routine to help maintain a sense of normalcy
    C. Focus on what works best for you and your family

Test Your Knowledge: Study Questions

Directions: Circle the letter corresponding to the correct response in each of the following.

1. If cancer cells are found in the lymph nodes, it is proof that the cancer has spread to other parts of the body.
   a. true
   b. false

2. Chemotherapy is a type of adjuvant therapy that involves the use of drugs that destroy only cancer cells throughout the body.
   a. true
   b. false

3. Radiation therapy to the local area of the breast is occasionally recommended following lumpectomy to destroy any remaining cancer cells.
   a. true
   b. false

4. A woman's menopausal status is important in planning for adjuvant therapy.
   a. true
   b. false

5. Only chemotherapy is known to have side effects as compared to radiation or hormonal therapy.
   a. true
   b. false

6. Chemotherapy can only be given into the vein.
   a. true
   b. false

7. It is up to the physician alone to evaluate the known and potential side effects of adjuvant therapy when making decisions about having treatment after surgery.
   a. true
   b. false

8. A rare side effect of radiation therapy is skin changes.
   a. true
   b. false

9. Most side effects from adjuvant therapy subside soon after the treatment has ended.
    a. true
    b. false

10. Fatigue, hair loss, and lowered resistance to infection are common side effects of chemotherapy drugs.
    a. true
    b. false

11. It is a good idea for a woman to wash the site with a strong soap before and after each radiation treatment session.
    a. true
    b. false

12. The bedside manner of the physician or the chemistry between patient and physician is important when choosing an oncologist for follow-up treatment
    a. true
    b. false

13. Help from friends and family members should not be necessary in order to manage household responsibilities while receiving adjuvant therapy.
    a. true
    b. false

14. Talking with women who have had chemotherapy usually is helpful.
    a. true
    b. false

15. Setting personal goals during adjuvant therapy is unrealistic since the experience varies so much.
    a. true
    b. false

4

Ongoing Recovery

This chapter explores some of the issues a woman and her partner face following adjuvant therapy with chemotherapy or radiation through the first year of recovery. This is a time when a woman will gradually return to her daily activities, while gaining back physical and emotional strength. It can be a period marked by enormous change and adjustment.

LINDA: *I had a great sense of relief. I was really, really lucky.*

CAROL: *I feel better than I felt before my surgery. I take better care of myself. Eat, we eat, I watch what we eat and exercise and all.*

NELLIE: *You know, it's a constant fear that you have to live with, sort of like every day of your life, you know. But then you have to try to divert your attention to other things, actually to help you through life.*

In the NYU study, the experiences of women and their partners were examined throughout the first year after diagnosis and the treatment of breast cancer. We found that cancer survival begins on the day of diagnosis and involves the active participation of a patient and her partner. That includes an awareness of needs and feelings, the promotion and protection of health, and a reentry into the mainstream in terms of both family and work roles.

The goals of this chapter are to help cancer survivors and their partners recognize emotional concerns and challenges; promote physical health and emotional well-being; continue and maintain a support network; and develop a plan for ongoing medical care.

RECOGNIZE EMOTIONAL CONCERNS
AND CHALLENGES

We begin by reflecting on some of the emotional concerns a woman may experience during this phase of recovery.

Some couples are surprised that the completion of therapy may involve ambivalence and separation anxiety from the health care system. Sometimes there is a sense of being abandoned as medical visits decrease or a feeling of vulnerability as therapy ends.

BOB: *After the second month and definitely by the third month we got into, this is the way it is for a couple of days and that's the way it's going to be. It really wasn't like you believed it to be. It was hard, though, there were times, those days were very tiring with the kids.*

LINDA: *I think once you've had cancer, whenever you have another pain in your body it's never quite the same again. You know, it's not that, "Oh, jeez, I'm getting old, there's a pain in my back." There's always that little voice in the back that says, "Uh oh, could it be back? Could it be elsewhere?"*

A diagnosis of breast cancer is followed by a roller coaster of emotions. In the 2 years after diagnosis and treatment, these initial feelings and emotions may be easily recalled at times of distress. Flashbacks about the experience may bring a composite of negative emotions. Considerable anxiety and emotional distress can also recur with the anniversary date of a diagnosis. This is a common experience for any individual who has suffered a loss in their life. These issues need to be understood before they can be put into perspective.

Women and their partners need to remember that during this ongoing recovery phase, they are regaining control over their lives, rather than losing it. The emphasis is on active participation in promoting health and well-being. Moving toward greater physical and emotional independence may create anxiety. Yet it is a testimony to a person's inner strength as a cancer survivor.

Taking control means asking questions and sharing information. Making a list of questions for physicians and nurses provides answers that help a woman manage her own care. Taking control also means expressing one's actual fears and feeling free to ask questions about lifestyle or changes in health.

Positive Attitude and Action

One way to develop a positive attitude is to reflect on the accomplishments one has achieved during one's journey to recovery. It's good to appreciate the progress already made. The cancer survivor has successfully dealt with many tough issues: selecting a physician and opting for surgery, recovering from either chemotherapy or radiation treatments. These are all enormous accomplishments.

CAROL: *I think I'm stronger than I thought I was. I thought if someone told me, "you will go through this," there's no way. Oh, I couldn't handle it. I would fall apart. I got through it and I feel good about that.*

Promoting Your Physical and Emotional Wellbeing

Fatigue can reduce both physical and emotional strength and lead to depression about the delay in returning to a more normal lifestyle.

CAROL: *I was very tired. Every day I would come home and take a nap. And it was just an exhausting, tired feeling I had. And it was such a depressing time.*

For other women, the experience of having breast cancer provides an opportunity to take a look at her lifestyle. It may provide an opportunity to make changes that will promote long-term health. It may be the time to slow down a previously unhealthy pace and to focus on ways of reducing stress and tension. This experience may be the impetus for a woman and her partner to live their lives as they truly want them to be.

CAROL: *Your life changes forever. At least mine did. You know, it's always there, but life is very important. I want to enjoy it. It's so precious and so short, and you just want to feel good, and your priorities change. Mine did.*

GEORGE: *We've always been savers, and we're always waiting for that big day you retire, but we decided that we wanted*

> *to enjoy ourselves a little bit more now. We're trying to do that. . . . I always wanted a sports car, so I bought a sports car this year. We did the deck last year. So those things, I mean, they're a bit materialistic, but they're also things that we postponed that maybe we shouldn't have.*

It's often helpful to know how other women have developed ways to incorporate healthy behaviors into their daily routines. New priorities may take more time and other things may have to be given up. But a woman's overall health and well-being should be priorities.

Many women find that work provides a source of satisfaction and stability in their lives. Carol had to take time off from work as a flight attendant, but soon returned, even though she was still tired from radiation treatments.

CAROL: *I had to take off during the radiation because I had to go Monday through Friday. My surgery was in April, and I had to complete the radiation, and I started as soon as I could. I went back to work in September of that year, 1991. And I was very nervous about going back. I didn't know if I could keep up. I was still tired.*

Nutrition

A healthy diet is also an important priority.

CAROL: *Initially after the surgery I got onto this very strict diet. I was very strict with myself, with my diet, and I started reading all kinds, whatever I could get my hands on about breast cancer and alternative therapies, alternative diets, very extreme. But now I'm more relaxed. Basically we eat a healthy, I feel a healthy, diet.*

GEORGE: *We try to eat less fat, less red meat, more fish. I think we eat out quite often, and when we do eat out I think I order fish every time or a vegetarian platter.*

GEORGE: *Carol comes home usually 7:30 to 8:30 at night. It's been a long day for her coming back from Europe or the west coast so I like to cook for her, and it's usually a pasta and we have our own herbs. We grow our own herbs.*

It is interesting to note that women athletes have a consistently lower incidence of breast cancer than nonathletes.

A healthy diet low in fat and high in fiber is recommended by the American Cancer Society. Moderate portions of salt-cured, smoked, and nitrite-cured foods, as well as dairy products and meats are also advised. Cruciferous vegetables, such as broccoli, cabbage, and cauliflower, are thought to have anti-breast cancer traits that deactivate the estrogen hormones. The hormones tend to support the growth of breast tumors.

Eating foods rich in vitamins A, C, and E may decrease the incidence of breast cancer.

As far as we know, obesity and high alcohol intake are risk factors for breast cancer. The goal is to maintain an optimal weight through a combination of both diet and exercise.

GEORGE: *Carol exercises more than I do.*

CAROL: *I go for my walks.*

GEORGE: *Yeah. I try a bit but I'm outside physically working every day. It's probably not enough, but that's what I do. And I watch what I eat. My weight is right for my age and my size.*

Hormonal Intake

It is controversial whether oral contraceptives or hormone replacement therapy are risk factors for breast cancer. The findings of recent studies are consistent with previous research about the relative risk of being diagnosed with breast cancer associated with estrogen replacement therapy (ERT) and hormone replacement therapy (HRT). The key finding suggests a small increase in the relative risk of being diagnosed with breast cancer associated with cyclic HRT, and a small increase in risk associated with duration of therapy. Importantly, continuous combined therapy, used by most women (80%) on HRT, did not show an increased risk for breast cancer (Schairer et al., 2000). A similar controversy exists in relation to the use of oral contraceptives (OC). Most of the overall risks reported lack statistical significance and do not warrant changes in practice. However, the use of ERT, HRT, and OC are generally contraindicated in women with known or suspected breast cancer or any estrogen-dependent cancer. Women should consult with their health care provider with specific questions about their individual situation.

> LINDA: *I did my own research and I really pursued my doctors, and I found that the medical community is changing their ideas around estrogen, and that maybe what's not right for one person may be okay for someone else. And so I have opted to go on it. I know what my risks are. I also know about my quality of life and what's important to me, and I weighed them, and I felt that the odds were in my favor, so it's something I have done. I'm also on progesterone with that, and it's really helped.*

Stress Reduction

Finally, one of the most important priorities for health and wellbeing is stress reduction. Women and their partners can spend some quiet time reflecting on those aspects of life that are sources of strength and pleasure, as well as identifying those that add stress. Some women value meditation as it provides an inner view of the self and a surfacing of previously unidentified feelings and needs. Writing down experiences offers a way to understand inner feelings and motivations. Other strategies for reducing stress include use of guided imagery, relaxation exercises, and yoga.

> CAROL: *Every day I would write about my feelings and about just how I felt physically, and it was just very painful at times. One very close friend, childhood friend, let me down because I think it was just too close for her, and she avoided me, and that was so painful.*

> LINDA: *You know, I think if I didn't have the children and worked full-time I definitely would have done some different things. And I probably would have kept a journal at night, although in the midst of chemotherapy I couldn't keep myself awake (laugh) at night. I was like, just start and I'd be out. But, you know, I love to cook and we have a big family room/kitchen, and we did a lot of that together as a family.*

BOB: *. . . we have little kids who monopolize 99% of your day
              so there really isn't a lot of choice. I always, and thank
              God for them, I mean, I'm active in their life so I've
              become part of their life.*

In the study of women and their partners at New York University
(NYU), couples talked about the benefit of reflecting on their experiences as a way to purge negative feelings and also to understand
the meaning of the illness in their lives. This was a personal activity that promoted greater self-awareness.

There are some very basic strategies to promote a better quality
of life:

- Learn to say "no" to things that are not in your best interest.
- Establish priorities.
- Recognize that humor is healthy and can improve your frame
  of mind.
- Focus on what you can and want to do, rather than on what
  you cannot do.
- Learn a new skill or hobby as a creative diversion and as a
  way to bolster good feelings.
- Reach out to others who are diagnosed with breast cancer.
- Take one day at a time and make the most of it.

CAROL: *I had a Bernie Siegel tape that helped me. Just any kind
              of relaxation tape and books were very important. I had
              to have a book that would really keep my interest, a real
              page turner; that's how I kept my mind off worrying.
              That really helped me a lot. I went to a place where they
              have nutritional food and exercise as a positive place,
              they call it a spa. It's kind of like a camp. I went there,
              and that was very positive, and it was good for me at the
              time just to be around people that are positive and
              healthy, and so I feel that's real important.*

NELLIE: *You try to deal with it, because I didn't have any family
              here, and so I prayed a lot, which I never did, and which
              actually reduced some of the stress.*

These are all very important suggestions to promote a sense of
wellbeing. Even so, it is not unusual to feel fine one day and a

little depressed the next. Healing physically and emotionally is not a linear, straightforward process. The uncertainty about recurrence can be a source of distress that persists for years after the completion of therapy.

MAINTAIN A SUPPORT NETWORK

After recovery, the need for support from the health care team will gradually lessen. However, a woman's progress should continue to be followed, working in partnership with her doctor and nurses.

CAROL: *I go for my checkups every 6 months. I would never miss them. But I block, I guess I block things out. It's like it never happened. I feel good.*

LINDA: *I make sure I go for those physicals. I make sure that I'm seen by someone probably every 4 months to have some sort of exam.*

If a woman feels anxious after completing therapy, it's helpful to share those concerns with the health care team. They can provide reassurance while helping her to feel more in control over any possible recurrences.

We'll talk now about how a woman and her partner can find continuing support from health care providers, family, and friends; cope with changing relationships; and find help through counseling or community resource groups.

Alterations in Relationships

Some women have the support of a partner and maybe children. Others must rely on the support of other significant persons in their lives. And just as a woman needs to be patient with herself during the recovery phase, it is important to understand the feelings of others.

CAROL: *Some people don't want to hear it. I can tell. And some people want to talk about it, and I, when it first happened, I didn't want anyone to know except family. . . . But we both have large families, and then I got to the point where that's selfish.*

GEORGE: *We had a family member that just went through a tough bout with cancer and did not make it. She died, and I felt like an outsider. I really felt that I was violating her space when I was visiting her. It was difficult for me not being a blood relative, if that should make the difference. But it was tough for me. And I think probably some of Carol's family members, maybe on my side, felt the same way. Violating.*

For significant others, the task of being supportive, while containing their own fears, may be very difficult. Some can cope with the impact of cancer sooner than others.

NELLIE: *Everybody needs people like that, you know, in their life, especially when you're going through a crisis. I think we all need people to help us.*

Being aware of verbal and nonverbal cues can help both individuals to determine when it is necessary to sit down and openly talk about their needs and feelings. These discussions may elicit feelings of sadness, isolation, helplessness, and even anger at the illness. In some relationships, the opposite of anger may be false cheer. It is only by recognizing each other's distress that feelings can be faced.

LINDA: *. . . what Bob was initially doing was saying, "no, no, no." I can do everything myself. And I knew he couldn't do everything himself. Just from an emotional standpoint he needed a break.*

BOB: *You have to be kind of realistic and give what needs to be given. For Linda, you know, we know each other really well. She knew that I needed some time so when she, because she'd do her chemo on Wednesday, sometimes by the weekend she'd be feeling okay. I would arrange something where I could go out and play with a group of my friends or go to New York. Once in a while I would, if we had somebody to stay over the house . . ., I'd escape for a day or two. So she knew what I needed. She knew when I was overloaded, when I needed something. She sometimes knew better than me.*

A woman and her partner may experience alterations in their relationships with family and friends. Although some people can be very supportive to a woman who has had a diagnosis of breast cancer, others may withdraw or disappear.

CAROL: *You never forget the certain friends that were just there and they would call all the time, offer to drive me to go for my radiation, and they were just there, and I knew they were there for me although I didn't, I drove myself every day. I was okay to do that. But just that support. But then you have other people that let you down, that you think they would be there, but they weren't. And then they come around later. I think because they were afraid.*

Kathleen Conway, who counsels cancer survivors, explains, "They may be afraid that they'll say something that will upset the person. They may be frightened of having to deal with talking to the person, their own feelings may come up. I think it's very scary when someone in the family has cancer, and it always brings up one's own fears or thoughts of mortality."

Carol was disappointed in a close friend who withdrew from her during her illness.

CAROL: *I told her how hurt I was and how 2 months have gone by and you never called. You know what I went through, and we went through so much together when my father passed away. She was there for me. And she really let me down, and I told her, and she listened, and I felt better that I had expressed myself.*

Reevaluate Feelings and Needs

It is helpful for women to reevaluate what they may be feeling or what they may need in regard to family, friends, and colleagues.

When a woman returns to work, her coworkers may either support her, avoid her, or wait for her cues on how to respond. Generally, it is helpful to resume good working relationships by planning in advance how to interact with coworkers. Some women choose to be very open with their coworkers, while others do not wish to focus on their cancer. It may also help to maintain work contacts during treatment and recovery. When able, a woman may want to stop by her job or plan lunch with coworkers. Even a simple phone call to the office can help to remain connected. It may also be important to ask an employer to educate employees about cancer, specifically that cancer is not a death sentence, is not contagious, and does not lessen the productivity of the survivor.

> LINDA: *There are certain things I need to just leave alone at this point. But I think it's up to you to make your colleagues more comfortable, your peers, your boss. You need to open up the lines of communication because they don't know, they're not sure whether they should talk about it, not talk about it.*

Likewise, there may be an array of responses from friends.

> LINDA: *I had some experiences with my immediate family you know, my parents, and that's when I talk about immediate family that weren't all as positive and supportive as I would have liked. And that was a shock and that wasn't easy to deal with, but I guess I did a shift and I told myself that my kids were going to be somewhere that I was going to look for support and I was going to look more to my friends who were there waiting in the wings ready and eager when I wanted them. And I think people who are trying to support a cancer patient have to realize that there are going to be times that you want it and times that you want people to back off. And they kind of have to be there. But I don't know. Bobby, what do you think?*

> BOB: *I felt pretty much the same way. None of our friends were the type that did not want to help. There weren't any that I know of that disappeared. But there were some people on the perimeter who knew of us through somebody else who you could tell when they came they were a little nervous or shy.*

> LINDA: *I called an aunt whom I'm particularly close to and I asked her if I could fly her up to Maine to be with us for at least 3 to 4 weeks. . . . But I think it was, it's easier for me to to deal with people on that level. Bobby had a tendency in some ways to say, "No, I can do it, I can do it."*

BOB: *I was really exhausted a lot of the time and I had to really push myself to let all of this help come in. My personality is "okay, let's grind through it." I'll get through it at my expense. And at times it was the wrong thing.*

A person who listens and validates individual needs and feelings is extremely important to healing and adjustment. Women and their partners often benefit from counseling as a resource to help them sort out feelings they may have.

BOB: *. . . there were days when I needed to talk to somebody. Not Lin, and not my kids or not my aunt. I needed to talk to somebody who didn't, who didn't know me. I needed to get something off my chest.*

LINDA: *. . . once I knew what I was going to do with chemotherapy, I was finished seeing doctors, now I was on a protocol, what we did do was, you know, we sought out some counseling. . . . You need to hear that from someone else. And someone who can help you sort through it who's not quite as emotionally involved, to say, "Yes, maybe you are doing the right thing by distancing yourself from a certain situation because now isn't the right time to deal with it." And I would highly recommend that to people because I think that wedges can come between you in your relationship if you aren't communicating and boy, oh boy, this isn't a time that you want that to happen.*

BOB: *I think counseling is great. And it's not something I discovered at this time but at the time I was very worried, I was as worried about the kids as I was about Lin. I didn't know what to worry about next.*

To regain health and quality of life means a woman needs to sometimes let go of negative emotions and focus on positive actions and attitudes.

If this is difficult to do and these feelings linger, it may be time to seek support from a psychologist, nurse therapist, or clinical social worker to help resolve recurrent emotional, marital, or family issues.

It's not uncommon for women who choose to participate in support groups to continue counseling. Kathleen Conway observes that "Sometimes they don't want to leave a group. There's a tremendous connection there. And they leave knowing that they live with a sort of fear of recurrence, that they want to do everything they can to stay healthy, to stay positive and to stay in charge, and that somehow the group can assist them in that, and more so than perhaps their family or their friends."

DEVELOP A PLAN FOR ONGOING MEDICAL CARE

A woman and her doctor should plan for regular follow-up visits once treatment is finished. If adjuvant therapy has been given, either the surgeon will oversee the follow-up care or refer care to the family physician, gynecologist, or internist.

Since 60% of all recurrences appear within the first 3 years after initial treatment, many doctors recommend an examination every 3 months for 1 year, then every 4 months for 2 years, and every 6 months for 5 years (see Table 4.1). If adjuvant therapy, such as tamoxifen, is continued, the medical oncologist may wish to participate in follow-up care.

Follow-Up Visits

For some women, the thought of a doctor's exam or follow-up tests creates anxiety. A return to the doctor's office or hospital, and perhaps seeing other patients, may evoke unpleasant memories and thoughts of recurrence. In coping with such anxiety, it's important for a woman to remember that she is a cancer survivor. Continued vigilance should reassure her of her making progress in regaining her health.

CAROL: *There were so many cancer survivors that I had no idea. I just thought cancer, it's just a matter of time and you're gone. But I met so many people that are doing well. They're healthy. They look healthy, and they have happy lives and that surprised me because I never really wanted to hear about cancer. . . . When I go for my checkups, I take my dog, my golden retriever, because twice after my surgery, the very next year I had to go for another biopsy.*

TABLE 4.1   Planning for Ongoing Care

- Sixty percent of all breast cancer recurrences appear within first 3 years after initial treatment
- Exams recommended:
  —every 3 months for 1 year
  —every 4 months for 2 years
  —every 6 months for 5 years
- Ongoing tamoxifen therapy may include medical oncologist follow-up

> *They found a lump on the other side. And of course I come out hysterical and she calms me down. She's just a dog but she calms me down.*

Annual mammograms are recommended for women that have been diagnosed with breast cancer. If a patient has had a lumpectomy with radiation therapy, an annual or more frequent mammogram of the affected breast will be determined by the radiation oncologist.

CAROL: *I go every 6 months, and I'm still nervous when I come out of there. It's such a good feeling that everything's okay. I still go through that: the fear. But it's not as much as it was.*

Self-Care

It is essential that women who have had breast cancer perform monthly self-examinations no matter what type of treatment they have had. Whether a lumpectomy or mastectomy, it is important to examine the original site to detect any signs of recurrence. It is equally important to examine the other breast to insure that no other cancer has developed. There are many videos or references that describe proper procedures for breast self-examination (see Table 4.2 and Figure 4.1).

It is important that any changes in the breast or presence of a lump be checked by a doctor. Although the majority of breast lesions are benign, accurate self-examinations are important, particularly with a history of a breast cancer.

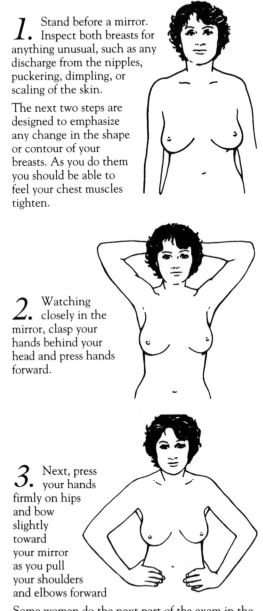

1. Stand before a mirror. Inspect both breasts for anything unusual, such as any discharge from the nipples, puckering, dimpling, or scaling of the skin.

The next two steps are designed to emphasize any change in the shape or contour of your breasts. As you do them you should be able to feel your chest muscles tighten.

2. Watching closely in the mirror, clasp your hands behind your head and press hands forward.

3. Next, press your hands firmly on hips and bow slightly toward your mirror as you pull your shoulders and elbows forward

Some women do the next part of the exam in the shower. Fingers glide over soapy skin, making it easy to concentrate on the texture underneath.

FIGURE 4.1   Breast self-examination.

Reproduced from American Institute for Cancer Research. (1993), *Questions and Answers About Breast Lumps and Breast Cancer,* copyright © 1993, American Institute for Cancer Research, Washington, DC. Reproduced by permission.

4. Raise your left arm. Use three or four fingers of your right hand to explore your left breast firmly, carefully and thoroughly. Beginning at the outer edge, press the flat part of your fingers in small circles, moving the circles slowly around the breast. Gradually work toward the nipple. Be sure to cover the entire breast. Pay special attention to the area between the breast and armpit, including the armpit itself. Feel for any unusual lump or mass under the skin.

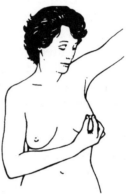

5. Gently squeeze the nipple and look for a discharge. Repeat the exam on your right breast.

6. Steps 4 and 5 should be repeated lying down. Lie flat on your back, left arm over your head and a pillow or folded towel under your left shoulder. This position flattens the breast and makes it easier to examine. Use the same circular motion described earlier. Repeat on your right breast.

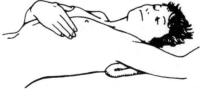

FIGURE 4.1 Breast self-examination *(continued)*.

TABLE 4.2 Monthly Self-Care

- Perform monthly self-exams
- Examine original site
- Examine other breast
- Follow correct technique for self-exam

Symptoms to Be Reported

It is a good idea to keep accurate, up-to-date records of all the medical care that has been received and other symptoms that are noted by self-evaluation. With a complete medical record, physicians can accurately evaluate present and future health needs. Report changes in the breast or scar, such as lumps, thickening, or pain in the breast. Also note pain in the hip, back, or other boney structure; problems related to the chest, such as coughing or hoarseness; symptoms related to the intestinal track if they persist beyond several days, such as nausea, vomiting, or diarrhea, and loss of weight or appetite; and changes in the menstrual cycle (see Table 4.3).

Ongoing recovery entails many physical and emotional changes. We hope the many issues we've covered in this chapter will help women and their partners on the road to a full recovery. We also hope that the information we have presented is helpful to health care providers in their work with breast cancer survivors. We learn from each other, and through our sharing, we each have the opportunity for personal growth.

TABLE 4.3 Symptoms to Be Reported

- Lumps, thickening, pain in the breast
- Pain in the hip, back, or other boney structure
- Problems related to the chest, such as coughing or hoarseness
- Symptoms related to the intestinal track if they persist beyond several days, such as nausea, vomiting, or diarrhea, and loss of weight or appetite
- Changes in the menstrual cycle

KNOWLEDGE REVIEW: ONGOING RECOVERY

Content Outline

This section includes an outline of the content of the chapter. It may be used as a review of the key points, or as a helpful aid to health professionals in preparing education materials for patients.

I. Emotional concerns and challenges
   A. A variety of emotions
      1. ambivalence
      2. separation anxiety from health care system
      3. sense of being abandoned
      4. feeling of vulnerability
   B. Emotions often fluctuate
      1. anxiety may recur with anniversary date of diagnosis
   C. Regaining control
      1. Active participation helpful
         a. ask questions
         b. express actual fears
         c. moving toward greater physical and emotional independence may create anxiety
   D. Develop positive attitude and action
      1. reflect on accomplishments
      2. appreciate progress
II. Promote physical and emotional well-being
   A. Recognize fatigue
   B. Have realistic expectations
   C. Examine lifestyle
   D. Establish priorities for a healthy lifestyle
      1. nutrition
      2. exercise
      3. control weight
      4. stress reduction to promote well-being
         a. meditation
         b. writing in journal
         c. reflecting on experiences
         d. relaxation tapes
   E. Healing physically and emotionally is not a linear, straightforward process
   F. Uncertainty about recurrence can be source of distress

III. Maintain a support network
    A. Need for support from health care team will gradually lessen
        1. progress should continue to be followed
        2. discuss anxiety after completing therapy
    B. Continued need for support from partner, children, and other significant persons
    C. Recognize needs and feelings of significant others
    D. Discuss needs and feelings with members of support network
    E. Withdrawal of friends and family members is not unusual
    F. Plan for return to work and how to interact with co-workers
        1. maintain work contacts during treatment and recovery
            a. lunch with co-workers
            b. phone calls
    G. Consider counseling as a resource
    H. Let go of negative emotions
    I. Utilize support groups
IV. Develop a plan for ongoing medical care
    A. Plan regular follow-up visits
        1. follow-up visits to doctor may create anxiety
            a. remember you are a survivor
        2. have regular mammogram
        3. perform breast self-examinations
        4. report
            a. any changes in breast
            b. pain in boney structures
            c. coughing or hoarseness
            d. digestive symptoms
            e. changes in menstrual cycle
        5. keep accurate, up-to-date record of all medical care received

Test Your Knowledge: Study Questions

Directions: Circle the letter corresponding to the correct response in each of the following.

1. Most women experience both positive and negative emotions when adjuvant therapy is completed.
    a. true
    b. false

2. Only when there is evidence of spread should a woman take extra care of her physical health after recovering from surgery and adjuvant therapy.
    a. true
    b. false

3. After treatment is completed, the anniversary date of diagnosis of breast cancer is often a time of celebration.
    a. true
    b. false

4. If a woman views herself as a cancer survivor rather than victim, it may improve her outlook and long-term wellbeing.
    a. true
    b. false

5. Exercise, proper nutrition, and recreation are more important during active treatment than during ongoing recovery from breast cancer.
    a. true
    b. false

6. Meditation and other forms of stress reduction are helpful in coping with the treatment and recovery phases of breast cancer.
    a. true
    b. false

7. Physical and emotional healing may continue gradually even after treatment is completed.
    a. true
    b. false

8. Women who try to manage without the support of others experience more anxiety and depression.
   a. true
   b. false

9. Professional counseling is sometimes helpful in dealing with the events and feelings associated with treatment and recovery for breast cancer.
   a. true
   b. false

10. Listening to her family's fears and concerns following her experience with breast cancer is important for family adjustment.
    a. true
    b. false

11. Returning to work should be delayed until a woman is finished with all treatment for breast cancer.
    a. true
    b. false

12. It is usually best if family roles and responsibilities during ongoing recovery return to normal as soon as possible.
    a. true
    b. false

13. Even when adjuvant therapy is completed, most women need to see the physician monthly for follow-up.
    a. true
    b. false

14. After a mastectomy, it is still important that breast self-examination be part of a woman's routine.
    a. true
    b. false

15. Once healing is complete it is not important for a woman to continue to examine her surgical site to note any changes in the way it looks or feels.
    a. true
    b. false

5

A Program of Research: Breast Cancer Education, Counseling, and Adjustment Among Patients and Partners

New diagnoses of breast cancer for 2000 were estimated at 183,000 (American Cancer Society, 2000). In the same year, 41,000 women were expected to die from the disease, often leaving behind families with growing children. More than 90% of women diagnosed and treated for the disease survive but often with a sense of uncertainty about their future, which in turn, affects adjustment.

While current surgical procedures for breast cancer are substantially less disfiguring than in previous years, and adjuvant therapy has been refined to allow better control of side effects, the treatment of breast cancer is not limited to medical management of a physical disease. Equally important are the psychological, informational, and support needs of the patient—and her family—which extend well beyond the first weeks following surgery. As unmet needs in any phase of the breast cancer experience may be carried over into subsequent phases, the protection of physical and emotional wellbeing and provision of social support must be expeditiously implemented to maximize the adjustment process.

PHASE I: PRELIMINARY STUDY

The women and health professionals interviewed for this book were all part of a larger research project conducted by nurse researchers at New York University. A preliminary study was designed to examine the effect of marital support and support from other adults on the emotional and physical adjustment of women with breast cancer and their partners (Hoskins, 1990–1994). The ability to function in usual roles and satisfaction with health care also were evaluated as predictors of adjustment. Data were obtained postsurgically at 7 to 10 days, 1 month, 2 months, 3 months, 6 months, and 1 year. The longitudinal design permitted the study of two different types of hypotheses: the relations between predictors and outcomes of adjustment at each phase, considered separately, and predictors from one time period to the adjustment outcomes at subsequent time periods.

Four hypotheses and one research question were examined: (1) less support in the marital relationship is related to more symptoms of emotional and physical maladjustment; (2) more support from adults other than the partner and from extended family is related to fewer symptoms of emotional and physical maladjustment; (3) more satisfaction with health care is related to a perception of better overall health status and more psychological wellbeing; (4) difficulty in performing life roles as a result of illness is related to more emotional and physical symptoms. The research question was: Do emotional and physical adjustment vary by breast conserving versus non-breast-conserving surgical groups and by positive versus negative node status groups?

A sample of 128 women and 121 partners met the inclusion criteria for missing data. At each data collection point, the respondents completed four standardized inventories: the Partner Relationship Inventory (Hoskins, 1988); the Psychosocial Adjustment to Illness Scale (Derogatis, 1983); the Profile of Adaptation to Life Clinical Scale (Ellsworth, 1981); the Self-Rated Health Subscale of the Multilevel Assessment Instrument (Lawton, Moss, Fulcomer, & Kleban, 1982), and a measure of current treatment and side effects to treatment (Hoskins, 1990).

The hypotheses were tested first for contemporaneous (zero time lag) relationships between predictor and outcome variables. Second, the hypotheses were tested for first-order lagged effects between predictor and outcome variables by canonical analyses that drew on the entire predictor set at each data collection point and on the outcome set at the immediately subsequent point. Third each hypothesis was evaluated in a canonical analysis that drew predictor variables from the 7- to 10-day postsurgery time and outcome variables from both the 6-months and 1-year points. The research question was examined by repeated measure analyses of variance.

Emotional adjustment could be predicted by marital support (perceived satisfaction with the partner's response to emotional and interaction needs) and by support from other adults (Hoskins et al., 1996a, 1996b). The relationships were significant at concurrent times, across contiguous times and predicting from the 7- to 10-day postsurgical phase to both the 6-month and 1-year end points. Physical adjustment was not predicted by support, but satisfaction with health care was predictive of overall health status. Functional status in vocational, domestic, and social roles was significantly related to emotional and physical adjustment at all phases with few exceptions. There was a significant difference in changes over time in physical symptoms between surgical groups and in overall health between node status groups. Women with positive nodes perceived their health status as lower at all times and had more psychological distress than women with negative nodes. Women and their partners experienced similar and yet different distress across the breast cancer experience. In some cases, partner adjustment was not as positive as that of the patients.

Four phases of emotional and physical adjustment were identified for both patients and partners: *diagnostic, postsurgical, adjuvant therapy,* and *ongoing recovery.* The specific needs associated with each phase were determined for each group. Needs were categorized as those related to: (a) physical well-being; (b) emotional well-being; (c) support; and (d) the health care system. The variation in intensity of needs in the four categories was documented across the four phases of the adjustment process and as they varied between patients and partners (Hoskins, 1995). At each of the four phases that emerged as critical markers in the adjustment process, satisfaction of needs related to social support and role performance promoted both physical and emotional adjustment.

The findings indicated the enormous importance of education, effective communication, and support in promoting physical and mental health among both women and their partners over time.

PHASE II: DEVELOPMENT OF THE STRUCTURED EDUCATIONAL INTERVENTION

Because a variety of adverse psychological and social factors impinged on the women who were diagnosed and treated for breast cancer and their partners, it was evident that state-of-the-art treatment for the illness needed to include educational and counseling interventions that addressed and ameliorated the substantial stressors involved both with the illness and its treatment. However, little was known from the literature about which modes of educational and counseling interventions would be most effective and for which categories of patients and family members, nor were the phase-specific needs of patients and families reported.

Using the extensive data base from the preliminary study, a series of four phase-specific, 30-minute videotapes were developed to provide a standardized research-based educational intervention for both patients and partners. The instructional videos, entitled *Journey To Recovery: For Women With Breast Cancer and Their Partners,* are designed to help women and men cope with the severe stress of the breast cancer experience. In the four-tape series, couples are guided through each phase of the disease and its treatment. Tape 1 helps couples cope with the *diagnosis.* Tape 2 walks couples through *recovery from surgery.* Tape 3 addresses the issues of *adjuvant therapy*—radiation, chemotherapy, or hormone treatment—, and tape 4 emphasizes the importance of the *ongoing recovery* process. The content of each videotape has a mental health focus and is organized under three main topics: (1) information required for making key treatment decisions, caring for self, and coping with the emotional impact of breast cancer; (2) methods and resources needed for developing a network of medical, informational, and supportive services; and (3) skills related to enhancing communication, managing stress, and developing a support system.

Many visuals are incorporated to convey the reality of the illness, yet are attuned to the emotional mindset of each patient and partner watching and learning. The many important points of each program are reinforced through effective real couple scenarios, visual effects, dynamic graphics, illustrations, and simple animation. Over the course of the four tapes, viewers learn from interview with a breast surgeon, a medical oncologist, two couples who participated in the initial research, and health care professionals.

As a set, the videotapes provide a standardized, research-based educational intervention program that can be used in a wide variety of treatment settings and followed by an opportunity to raise individual concerns with a clinical nurse oncologist, physician, or breast service coordinator.

PHASE III: PILOT STUDY AND START-UP OF A RANDOMIZED CLINICAL TRIAL

Phase III consisted of an initial pilot study to test the feasibility of a confirmatory randomized clinical trial. The aim was to implement and compare the effectiveness of the three components of the intervention. The four interventions formed a tiered or incremental approach to disease management of breast cancer at each of the four phases identified in Phase I.

The crisis intervention model developed by Morely, Messick, and Aguilera (1967), combined with the coping model by Lazarus (1966), provided the theoretic framework for the intervention components. According to the crisis intervention model, the degree and character of psychosocial distress experienced by breast cancer patients and their partners depend on their specific perceptions of the meaning of the stressful situation, previous exposure to similar stress, adaptiveness of their coping mechanisms, and adequacy of support systems (Aguilera, 1998; Capone, Good, Westie, & Jacobson, 1980; Parad & Parad, 1990).

Crises frequently result from lack of balancing factors that maximize adjustment as attempts are made to return to a state of equilibrium following a stressful event (Aguilera, 1998). Women diagnosed with breast cancer, and their partners, can be regarded as being at high risk for a situational crisis. The focus of the model is on crisis prevention by maximizing physical adjustment and emotional adjustment, role performance, perceived social support, and overall health status. The model provided the theoretic framework for the telephone counseling sessions at the four phases in the illness-recovery period.

Consistent with this approach, informational interventions help patients see how they can assume an active role in treatment and maintaining control (Cohen & Lazarus, 1979). Four essential types of information maximize adjustment: (1) the nature of the disease and the medical reasons for initiating specific treatments; (2) the potential medical procedures; (3) the expected side effects; and (4) the strategies that can be used to cope with upcoming threats (Cohen & Lazarus, 1979; Derdiarian, 1987a, 1987b, 1989; Hoskins & Haber, 1997).

INTERVENTIONS

- A first group received the currently accepted *disease management (DM)* of breast cancer—an intervention all four groups received.
- A second group received DM and the *structured education by videotape* produced in Phase II.
- A third group received DM, the *education by videotape,* and *telephone counseling.*

Structured Education by Videotape

The structured education component of the intervention consists of the four phase-specific videotapes. As noted, the content of each videotape was organized under three topics: (1) health relevant information; (2) skills training; and (3) psychosocial support. The intervention was conducted by a research fellow, that is, a doctoral student who was trained to administer the intervention, including the pretest and posttest, an evaluation form for the intervention, and a battery of instruments for evaluating social support and various dimensions of adjustment.

Telephone Counseling

The 30-minute phase-specific telephone counseling is an individualized intervention designed to enhance the client's belief that the counselor will be able to help, a necessity if treatment goals are to be accomplished in a short time (Bellack & Small, 1965). The telephone counseling intervention consists of the four individual phase-specific telephone counseling sessions for each patient and partner. The sessions were conducted by a second research fellow trained in individualized telephone counseling approaches. The fellow also was trained to administer the evaluation form for the intervention and the battery of instruments for evaluating social support and various dimensions of adjustment. The setting for the intervention was the home. A telephone audiotape player was used to record each session for supervision and validation.

Structured Education + Telephone Counseling

The third component of the intervention combined in entirety the structured education with the brief telephone counseling. The sessions were conducted by a third research fellow trained to administer the intervention, the pretest and posttest, the evaluation form, and the battery of instruments for evaluating social support and adjustment.

Prior to the accrual of patients and partners for the pilot study, (a) the Education and Telephone Counseling Training Manual was developed as a guide for all aspects of the protocols; (b) research fellows were trained in the intervention components; (c) evaluation forms for obtaining data on process variables were constructed; and (d) pretests and posttests for the structured education were developed.

The required nonprobability sample of 12 patient–partner pairs was accrued, four pairs for each of the three intervention components. The intervention components were administered to patients and partners separately at each of the four phases identified in the preliminary study (diagnosis, postsurgery, adjuvant therapy, and ongoing recovery), and data were collected according to the research design.

The feasibility of a confirmatory clinical trial was demonstrated by the pilot study, thus providing support for examining the unique contribution of phase-specific structured education and telephone counseling to the ongoing process of adjustment among patients and the "partner" identified as the person most intimately involved in the events related to the illness and treatment. The strengths of the proposed clinical trial included: (a) a theoretic approach that was well delineated; (b) interventions that were research based and phase specific; (c) outcomes that were well conceptualized and operationalized by valid and reliable measures; and (d) inclusion of primary partners in interventions and assessment of adjustment. The high retention rates of patient–partner pairs achieved in the preliminary study were duplicated in the pilot study, data were obtained and used for estimation of sample size and power for the clinical trial, and issues relevant to data collection and management were identified and addressed. The feasibility of a full confirmatory randomized clinical trial was demonstrated.

References

Aguilera, D. C. (1998). *Crisis intervention: Theory and methodology* (8th ed.). St. Louis: C. V. Mosby.

American Cancer Society. (1998). Cancer statistics 1998. *CA: A cancer journal for clinicians, 48*(1), 10–31.

American Cancer Society. (2000). Cancer statistics 2000. *CA: A cancer journal for clinicians, 50*(1), 7–33.

Baron, R. H. (1999). Sentinel lymph node biopsy in breast cancer and the role of the oncology nurse. *Clinical Journal of Oncology Nursing, 3*(1), 17–22.

Bellack, L., & Small, L. (1965). *Emergency psychotherapy and brief psychotherapy.* New York: Grune & Stratton.

Capone, M. A., Good, R. S., Westie, K. S., & Jacobson, A. F. (1980). Psychosocial rehabilitation of gynecologic oncology patients. *Archives of Physical Medicine and Rehabilitation, 61,* 128–132.

Cohen, F., & Lazarus, R. C. (1979). Coping with the stress of illness. In G. C. Stone, F. Cohen, & N. E. Nadler (Eds.), *Health psychology* (pp. 247–254). San Francisco: Jossey-Bass.

Derdiarian, A. K. (1987a). Informational needs of recently diagnosed cancer patients. Part 1: A theoretical framework. *Cancer Nursing, 10,* 107–115.

Derdiarian, A. K. (1987b). Informational needs of recently diagnosed cancer patients. Part II: Method and description. *Cancer Nursing, 10,* 156–163.

Derdiarian, A. K. (1989). Effects of information on recently diagnosed cancer patients' and spouses' satisfaction with care. *Cancer Nursing, 12,* 285–292.

Derogatis (1983). *The Psychosocial Adjustment to Illness Scale.* Towson, MD: Clinical Psychometric Research.

Ellsworth, R. (1981). *Profile of Adaptation to Life Clinical Scale.* Palo Alto, CA: Consulting Psychologists Press.

Gross, R. E. (1998). Current issues in the surgical treatment of early stage breast cancer. *Clinical Journal of Oncology Nursing, 2*(2), 55–63.

Hortobagyi, G. N. (1998). Treatment of breast cancer. Review of Drug Therapy. *New England Journal of Medicine, 339,* 974–984.

Hoskins, C. N. (1988). *The partner relationship inventory.* Palo Alto, CA: Consulting Psychologists Press.

Hoskins, C. N. (1990–1994). Patterns of adjustment among women with breast cancer and their partners (funded by the Walter Langer Foundation).

Hoskins, C. N. (1990). *The Breast Cancer Treatment Response Inventory.* Unpublished measure of treatment and side effects.

Hoskins, C. N. (1995). Adjustment to breast cancer in couples. *Psychological Reports, 77,* 435–454.

Hoskins, C. N., Baker, S., Bohlander, J., Bookbinder, M., Budin, W., Ekstrom, D., Knauer, C., Maislin, G., & Sherman, D. (1996a). Social support and patterns of adjustment to breast cancer. *Journal of Scholarly Inquiry for Nursing Practice: An International Journal, 10*(2), 99–123.

Hoskins, C. N., Baker, S., Bohlander, J., Bookbinder, M., Budin, W., Ekstrom, D., Knauer, C., Maislin, G., & Sherman, D. (1996b). Adjustment among spouses of women with breast cancer. *Journal of Psychosocial Oncology, 14*(1), 41–69.

Hoskins, C. N., & Haber, J. (1997). *Journey to recovery: For women with breast cancer and their partners.* A four-part videotape series filmed by Euro Pacific Film and Video Productions, Inc. (L. Moss, Director). Princeton, NJ: Films for the Humanities and Sciences.

Lawton, M. P., Moss, M. S., Fulcomer, M., & Kleban, M. H. (1982). A research and service oriented Multilevel Assessment Instrument. *Journal of Gerontology, 37,* 91–99.

Morely, W. E., Messick, J. M., & Aguilera, D. C. (1967). Crisis: Paradigms of intervention. *Journal of Psychiatric Nursing, 5,* 537.

National Comprehensive Cancer Network (NCCN) & American Cancer Society (ACS). (1999). *Breast Cancer Treatment Guidelines for Patients* (pp. 1–38).

Parad, H. J., & Parad, L. G. (1990). Crisis intervention: An introductory overview. In H. J. Parad & L. G. Parad (Eds.), *Crisis intervention: The practitioner's sourcebook for brief therapy* (pp. 1–66). Milwaukee, WI: Family Service America.

Parker, S. L., Tong, T., Bolden, S., & Wingo, P. A. (1997). Cancer statistics, 1997. *CA: A cancer journal for clinicians, 47,* 5–27.

Powles, T. J. (1999). A review of results from the NSABP and Royal Marsden Chemoprevention Trials. *Primary Care & Cancer* (Suppl. 2), 21–23.

Schairer, C., Lubin, J., Troisi, R., Sturgeon, S., Brinton, L., & Hoover, R. (2000). Menopausal estrogen-progestin replacement therapy and breast cancer risk. *Journal of the American Medical Association, 283,* 485–491.

APPENDIX

Cancer Resources in the United States

American Association for
   Cancer Education
P.O. Box 601
Smellville, GA 30078-0601
404-329-7612
gkrawiec@cancer.org

American Cancer Society
1599 Clifton Road, NE
Atlanta, GA 30329-4251
404-329-7623 (patient services)
800-ACS-2345
www.cancer.org

American College of Radiology
1391 Preston White Drive
Reston, VA 22091

American Institute for Cancer
   Research
1759 R Street, NW
Washington, DC 20009
800-843-8114 (nutrition hotline,
   publications department)

American Society of Plastic
   and Reconstructive
   Surgeons
444 East Algonquin Road
Arlington Heights, IL 60005
800-635-0635
www.plasticsurgery.org

Association of Community
   Cancer Centers
11600 Nebel Street
Suite 201
Rockville, MD 20852
301-984-9496
www.accc-cancer.org

Cancer Care, Inc.
275 Seventh Avenue
New York, NY 10001
212-302-2400
800-813-HOPE
www.cancercare.org

From Cancer resources in the United States (1999). *Oncology Nursing Forum, 26*(9), 1525-1538.

CancerNet
NCI International Cancer
  Information Center
9030 Old Georgetown Road
Bethesda, MD 20814-1519
cancernet.nci.nih.gov

Cancer Hope Network
Two North Road, Suite A
Chester , NJ 07930
877-HOPENET
www.cancerhopenetwork.org

Cancer Information Service
National Cancer Institute
800-4-CANCER

**Cancer Recovery Foundation
  of America**
P.O. Box 238
Hershey, PA 17033
800-238-6479
www.wellness.net

Cancer Services on the Internet
http://www.meds.com/

Coping
Media America, Inc.
P.O. Box 682268
Franklin, TN 37068-2268
614-790-2400
Copingmag@aol.com

Corporate Angel Network, Inc.
Westchester County Airport
One Loop Road
White Plains, NY 10604
914-328-1313
www.corpangelnetwork.org

**Gillette Women's Cancer
  Connection**
800-688-9777
www.gillettecancerconnect.org

Johanna's of Albany Ltd.
4 Executive Park Drive
Albany, NY 12203
518-459-2252

Look Good . . . Feel Better
1101 17th Street, NW
Suite 300
Washington, DC 20036
800-395-LOOK

LymphEdema Foundation
P.O. Box 834
San Diego, CA 92014-0834
800-LYMPH-DX

Make Today Count
1235 East Cherokee
Springfield, MO 65804-2262
417-885-2273
800-432-2273

**Mary-Helen Mautner
  Project for Lesbians
  with Cancer**
1707 L Street, NW, Suite 500
Washington, DC 20036
202-332-5536

**National Alliance of Breast
  Cancer Organizations**
9 East 37th Street, 10th Floor
New York, NY 10016
888-80-NABCO
www.nabco.org

National Black Leadership Initiative on Cancer
6120 Executive Boulevard South
Suite 320
Bethesda, MD 20892
301-496-8589
fj121@nih.gov

National Breast Cancer Coalition
1707 L Street NW
Suite 1060
Washington, DC 20036
202-296-7477
www.natlbcc.org

National Cancer Survivors Day Foundation, Inc.
P.O. Box 682285
Franklin, TN 37068-2285
615-794-3006
www.NCSDF.org

National Coalition for Cancer Research
426 C Street NE
Washington, DC 20002
202-544-1880

National Coalition for Cancer Survivorship
1010 Wayne Avenue
Silver Spring, MD 20910
877-NCCS-YES
www.cansearch.org

National Hispanic Leadership Initiative on Cancer
South Texas Health Research Center
University of Texas Health Sciences Center at San Antonio
7703 Floyd Curl Drive
San Antonio, TX 78284-7791
210-567-7826

National Lymphedema Network
2211 Post Street
Suite 404
San Francisco, CA 94115-3427
800-541-3259
www.lymphnet.org

National Surgical Adjuvant Breast and Bowel Project
NSABP Operations Center
East Commons Professional Building, Fifth Floor
Four Allegheny Center
Pittsburgh, PA 15212-5234
412-330-4600

Office of Minority Health Resource Center
U.S. Department of Health and Human Services
P.O. Box 37337
Washington, DC 20013-7337
800-444-6472
www.omhrc.gov

PDQ (Physician Data Query)
NCI International Cancer
  Information Center
9030 Old Georgetown Road
Bethesda, MD 20814-1519
800-4-CANCER (patient
  information)
cancernet.nci.nih.gov

**R.A. Bloch Cancer
  Foundation, Inc.
The Cancer Hotline**
4400 Main Street
Kansas, MO 64111
816-932-8453

**Susan G. Komen Breast
  Cancer Foundation**
5005 LBJ Freeway, Suite 250
Dallas, TX 75244
800-I'M AWARE or
  800-462-9273
  (national helpline)

Wellness Community
2716 Ocean Park Boulevard
Suite 1040
Santa Monica, CA 90405

310-314-2555 or 513-794-1116
888-793-WELL

**Y-ME National Breast Cancer
  Organization**
212 W. Van Buren, Fifth Floor
Chicago, IL 60607-3908
800-221-2141 (toll-free hotline,
  24 hours)
800-986-9505 (Hispanic hotline,
  24 hours)
www.Y-ME.org

YWCA
YWCA of the U.S.A. Encore
  Program
Office of Women's Health
  Initiatives
624 Ninth Street, NW,
  Third Floor
Washington, DC 20001
202-628-3636

Answers to "Test Your Knowledge" Questions

ANSWERS TO CHAPTER 1 STUDY QUESTIONS

1. a
2. b
3. b
4. a
5. b
6. a
7. a
8. a
9. b
10. b
11. a
12. a
13. b
14. b
15. a

ANSWERS TO CHAPTER 2 STUDY QUESTIONS

1. b
2. a
3. b
4. a
5. b

6. a
7. a
8. b
9. b
10. a
11. b
12. b
13. b
14. b
15. a

ANSWERS TO CHAPTER 3 STUDY QUESTIONS

1. b
2. b
3. b
4. a
5. b
6. b
7. b
8. b
9. a
10. a
11. b
12. a
13. b
14. a
15. b

ANSWERS TO CHAPTER 4 STUDY QUESTIONS

1. a
2. b
3. b
4. a
5. b
6. a
7. a

8. a
9. a
10. a
11. b
12. b
13. a
14. a
15. b

Index

ACS, *see* American Cancer Society
(ACS)
Adjuvant therapy
definition of, 47
factors related to, 51
indications for, 53
information about
cancer resources, contact
information, 103–106
obtaining, 54–56
introduction to, *viii*, 47
knowledge review and study
questions about, 64–69
physical and emotional health,
management of, 56–57
goal setting, strategies for, 63
infections, management of, 58
menopause-like symptoms,
management of, 60–61
nutrition and, 58–59
rest and activity, balancing of,
59–60
side effects, management of,
57–58
stress, management and, 61–63
types of
chemotherapy, 48–52
hormone therapy, 52–53,
74–75
introduction to, 48
radiation therapy, 53–54, 58
tamoxifen and, 52–54, 58
Aguilera, D. C., 95, 99–100

American Association for Cancer
Education, contact information,
103
American Cancer Society (ACS)
community resource programs, 21
contact information, 103
diet recommendations, 74
Reach to Recovery program,
21, 38
statistical data, 91, 99, *vii*
treatment guidelines, 51, 100
American College of Radiology,
contact information, 103
American Institute for Breast Cancer
Research, 84–85
American Institute for Cancer
Research, contact information,
103
American Society of Plastic and
Reconstructive Surgeons,
contact information, 103
Ashikari, Roy, *viii*, 10, 15, 37
Association of Community Cancer
Centers, contact information,
103

Baker, S., 100
Baron, R. H., 12, 99
Bellack, L., 96, 99
Bohlander, J., 100
Bolden, S., 101
Bookbinder, M., 100
Budin, W., 100

Cancer Care, Inc., contact information, 103
Cancer Hope Network, contact information, 104
Cancer Hotline, The, contact information, 106
Cancer Information Service, contact information, 104
Cancer Recovery Foundation of America, contact information, 104
Cancer Services on the Internet, contact information, 104
CancerNet, contact information, 104
Capone, M. A., 95, 99
Cartwright-Alcarese, Frances, *viii*
Center for Hope (Connecticut), 16
Chemotherapy, 48–52; *see also* Adjuvant therapy
Cohen, F., 95–96, 99
Conversations with survivors and partners
 Bob, *viii*, 1, 16, 18, 35–37, 55, 59–60, 62–63, 71, 76, 78, 80–81
 Carol, *viii*, 1, 3, 8, 12, 17, 19–20, 28, 33, 37, 54, 59, 61, 70, 72–77, 79, 82–83
 George, *viii*, 1, 19, 28, 35, 59, 61, 72–74, 78
 Linda, *viii*, 1, 3, 6, 8, 13, 15–18, 28–31, 33–38, 48, 55–62, 70–71, 75, 77–78, 80–81
 Nellie, *viii*, 1, 3, 12, 17, 28, 30, 53–54, 61, 70, 76, 78
Conway, Kathleen, 16, 18–19, 34, 56, 62–63, 79
Coping (Media America, Inc.), contact information, 104
Coping skills
 adjuvant therapy, understanding, *viii*, 47–69
 diagnosis and, *vii*, 1–27
 ongoing recovery and, *viii*, 70–90
 surgery recovery and, *vii*, 28–46
Corporate Angel Network, Inc., contact information, 104

Derdiarian, A. K., 96, 99
Diagnosis of breast cancer, coping with
 breast cancer
  facts about, 2–4
  introduction to, *vii*, 1–2
  risk factors, 5
  stages of, 8–9
  types of, 5–8
 diagnostic methods, 4–10
 health care resources
  contact information, 103–106
  identification of, 20–22
 knowledge review of and study questions about, 23–27
 perceptions, emotions, and concerns and, 16–17
 stress management and, 17–20
 treatments, surgical, 10–16

Ekstrom, D., 100
Ellsworth, R., 92, 100
Euro-Pacific Film and Video Productions, *viii*

Fulcomer, M., 92, 100

Gillette Women's Cancer Connection, contact information, 104
Good, R. S., 95, 99
Gross, R. E., 10, 100

Haber, J., 96, 100
Hormone therapy, 52–53, 74–75; *see also* Adjuvant therapy
Hortobagyi, G. N., 3, 51–52, 100
Hoskins, Carol Noll, *vii–viii*, 92–93, 96, 100

Instruments, measurement, *see* Inventories, standardized
Inventories, standardized
 measure of current treatment and side effects to treatment (unnamed), 92–98
 Partner Relationship Inventory, 92–98

Profile of Adaptation to Life Clinical Scale, 92–98
Psychological Adjustment to Illness Scale, 92–98
Self-Rated Health Subscale of the Multilevel Assessment Instrument, 92–98

Jacobson, A. F., 95, 99
Johanna's of Albany Ltd., contact information, 104
Journey to Recovery: For Women with Breast Cancer and Their Partners (video publication), *vii–viii*, 94–95

Kleban, M. H., 92, 100
Kloos, Elaine, 4
Knauer, C., 100
Knowledge review and study questions
adjuvant therapy, 47–69
answers, 107–109
diagnosis, coping with, 23–27
ongoing recovery and, 87–90
surgery, recovery from and coping with, 42–46
Kowalski, Mildred Ortu, *viii*

Lawton, M. P., 92, 100
Lazarus, R. C., 95–96, 99
Look Good . . . Feel Better, contact information, 104
LymphEdema Foundation, contact information, 104

Maislin, G., 100
Make Today Count, contact information, 104
Mary-Helen Mautner Project for Lesbians with Cancer, contact information, 104
McNeil, George, *viii*
Measurement instruments, *see* Inventories, standardized
Medical facilities
Center for Hope (Connecticut), 16

Monmouth Medical Center (New Jersey), 4, 20, 36
New York University, *see* New York University, four-year study on breast cancer
St. Agnes Hospital (White Plains, New York), 37, 51
Messick, J. M., 95, 100
Mittleman, Abraham, *viii*, 51–52
Monmouth Medical Center (New Jersey), 4, 20, 36
Morely, W. E., 95, 100
Moss, Linda, *viii*
Moss, M. S., 92, 100

National Alliance of Breast Cancer Organizations
contact information, 104
information about, 21
National Black Leadership Initiative on Cancer, contact information, 105
National Breast Cancer Coalition, contact information, 105
National Cancer Survivor Day Foundation, Inc., contact information, 105
National Coalition for Cancer Research, contact information, 105
National Coalition for Cancer Survivorship, information about, 105
National Comprehensive Cancer Network (NCCN), 51–52, 100
National Hispanic Leadership Initiative on Cancer, contact information, 105
National Lymphedema Network, contact information, 105
National Surgical Adjuvant Breast and Bowel Project (NSABP)
contact information, 105
information about, 72
NCCN, *see* National Comprehensive Cancer Network (NCCN)

New York University, four-year study on breast cancer
 conversations with survivors and partners, *see* Conversations with survivors and partners
 descriptions of, 2, 17, 28–33, 56–62, 70, 76, 92
 interventions, 96–98
 introduction to, *vii–viii*, 91
 phase one, preliminary study, 92–93
 phase three, pilot study and clinical trial, 95–96
 phase two, structured educational intervention, 94–95
NSABP, *see* National Surgical Adjuvant Breast and Bowel Project (NSABP)
Nutrition, impact of, 58–59, 73–74

Office of Minority Health Resource Center, contact information, 105
Ongoing recovery
 emotional concerns and challenges
  hormone intake and, 74–75
  introduction to, *viii*, 71–72
  nutrition and, 73–74
  positive attitude and actions, 72
  promoting physical and emotional well-being, 72–73
  stress reduction and, 75–77
 introduction to, 70
 knowledge review and study questions about, 87–90
 ongoing medical care and
  breast self-examinations and, 84–86
  follow-up doctor visits, 82–83
  introduction to, 82
  self-care and, 83–86
  symptoms to report, 86
 support networks and
  introduction to, 77
  reevaluation of feelings and needs, 79–82
  relationships, alterations in, 77–79

Panke, Joan, *viii*
Parad, H. J., 95, 100
Parad, L. G., 95, 100
Parker, S. L., 101
Partner Relationship Inventory, 92–98
Partners and survivors, *see* Survivors and partners
PDQ, *see* Physician Data Query (PDQ), contact information
Physician Data Query (PDQ), contact information, 106
Powles, T. J., 52, 101
Profile of Adaptation to Life Clinical Scale, 92–98
Psychological Adjustment to Illness Scale, 92–98
Psychological recovery, strategies to promote, 33–39, 103–106

R. A. Bloch Cancer Foundation, Inc., contact information, 106
Rabinowitz, Barbara, 20–21, 36–37, 40
Radiation therapy, 53–54, 58; *see also* Adjuvant therapy
Reach to Recovery program, 21, 38; *see also* American Cancer Society (ACS)
Recovery
 ongoing, *see* Ongoing recovery
 surgery, recovery from, *see* Surgery, recovery from and coping with
Research, programs of
 introduction to, 91
 New York University, four-year study
  interventions, 96–98
  introduction to, 91
  phase one, preliminary study, 92–93
  phase three, pilot study and clinical trial, 95–96
  phase two, structured educational intervention, 94–95
Risk factors for breast cancer, 5

Self-examinations, 84–86
Self-Rated Health Subscale of the
    Multilevel Assessment
    Instrument, 92–98
Sherman, D., 100
Sherman, Deborah, *viii*
Small, L., 96, 99
St. Agnes Hospital (White Plains,
    New York), 37, 51
Stages of breast cancer, 8–9
Standardized inventories, *see*
    Inventories, standardized
Stress management, 17–20, 61–63, 75–77
Study questions, *see* Knowledge
    review and study questions
Support networks, 77–82
Surgery, recovery from and coping
    with
    family changes, management of,
        39–41
    feelings after surgery, recognition
        of, 29–33
    introduction to, *vii*, 28–29
    knowledge review and study
        questions about, 42–46
    psychological recovery, strategies to
        promote
        community resources and, 38–39,
            103–106
        development of, 33–35
        introduction to, 33
        support systems, creation of,
            35–38
    social roles, management of,
        39–41
    summary of, 41

Survivors and partners, conversations
    with
    Bob, *viii*, 1, 16, 18, 35–37, 55,
        59–60, 62–63, 71, 76, 78,
        80–81
    Carol, *viii*, 1, 3, 8, 12, 17,
        19–20, 28, 33, 37, 54, 59,
        61, 70, 72–77, 79,
        82–83
    George, *viii*, 1, 19, 28, 35, 59, 61,
        72–74, 78
    Linda, *viii*, 1, 3, 6, 8, 13,
        15–18, 28–31, 33–38,
        48, 55–62, 70–71, 75,
        77–78, 80–81
    Nellie, *viii*, 1, 3, 12, 17, 28, 30, 53–54,
        61, 70, 76, 78

Tamoxifen, 52–54, 58; *see also*
    Adjuvant therapy
Test your knowledge questions, *see*
    Knowledge review and study
    questions
Therapy, adjuvant, *see* Adjuvant
    therapy
Tong, T., 101

Wellness Community, contact
    information, 106
Westie, K. S., 95, 99
Wingo, P. A., 101

Y-ME National Breast Cancer
    Organization, contact
    information, 106
YWCA, contact information, 106

⑤ Springer Publishing Company

Preventing and Managing Osteoporosis

Sarah Hall Gueldner, DSN, FAAN, **M. Susan Burke,** MD
Helen Smiciklas-Wright, PhD, Editors

This book will raise awareness and inform health professionals about this often preventable and treatable disease. Written by a team of authors from medicine, nursing, nutrition, exercise physiology, and physical therapy, the volume provides an overview of the disease process—discussing its epidemiology, strategies for prevention and treatment, as well as the clinical implications of osteoporosis across disciplines.

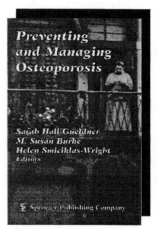

Contents:
- Epidemiology: The Magnitude of Concern
- Living With Osteoporosis: The Personal Experience
- Nutritional Considerations
- Exercise: A Prescription for Osteoporosis?
- Bone Remodeling and the Development of Osteoporosis
- Patient Identification and Evaluation
- Therapeutic Strategies for Prevention and Treatment
- Osteoporosis and Fall Prevention
- Relief of Pain
- Adapting Clothing to Accommodate Changes in the Body
- Target Groups for Prevention and Early Detection
- Clinical Implications Across Disciplines

2000   216pp.   0-8261-1318-4   hard

536 Broadway, New York, NY 10012 • (212)431-4370 • Fax: (212)941-7842
Order Toll-Free: (877) 687-7476 • *www.springerpub.com*

SP *Springer Publishing Company*

Palliative Care Nursing
Quality Care to the End of Life

Marianne LaPorte Matzo, PhD, RN, GNP, CS
Deborah Witt Sherman, PhD, RN, ANP, CS, Editors

"This text will be recognized as a foundation for nursing education. The authors ... are recognized leaders in palliative nursing education....The text is a comprehensive approach spanning the traditional to complementary treatments."
—**Betty Rolling Ferrell**, RN, PhD, FAAN, from the Foreword

This book provides essential information on the best practices for quality care at the end of life. It is organized around the 15 competencies in palliative care developed by the American Association of Colleges of Nursing. The book combines holistic, humanistic caring with aggressive management of pain and symptoms. Comprehensive clinical content is combined with curriculum guidelines for educators. This book is for students and educators at all levels of nursing education, and for practicing nurses working with the terminally ill.

Contents: **Part 1. Holistic Aspects of Palliative Care** • Spiritually and Culturally Competent Palliative Care, *D.W. Sherman* • Holistic Integrative Therapies in Palliative Care, *C. Mariano* • **Part 2. Social Aspects of Palliative Care** • Death and Society, *M. Bookbinder & M. Kiss* • The Nurse's Roles in Interdisciplinary and Palliative Care, *L.M. Krammer, et al.* • Ethical Aspects of Palliative Care, *J.K. Schwarz* • Legal Aspects of Palliative Care, *G.C. Ramsey* • **Part 3. Psychological Aspects of Dying** • Communicating With Seriously Ill and Dying Patients, Their Families, and Their Health Care Providers, *K.O. Perrin* • Caring for Families: The Other Patient in Palliative Care, *S.K. Goetschius* • Loss, Suffering, Bereavement, and Grief, *M.L. Potter* • **Part 4. Physical Aspects of Palliative Care** • Symptom Management in Palliative Care, *M.K. Kazanowski* • Pain Assessment and Management in Palliative Care, *N. Coyle and M. Layman-Goldstein* • Peri-Death Nursing Care, *M.L. Matzo* • Appendixes

2001   520pp.   0-8261-1384-2   hard

536 Broadway, New York, NY 10012 • **(212)431-4370** • **Fax: (212)941-7842**
Order Toll-Free: (877) 687-7476 • *www.springerpub.com*